Managing Chronic Diseases: A Practical Guide to Daily Control of Diabetes, Hypertension, and Musculoskeletal Issues

Self-Management and Prevention Tools to Improve Quality of Life and Reduce Symptoms

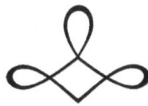

Dr. Emily Roberts

Table of Contents

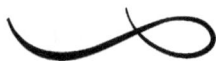

Chapter 1: Understanding Chronic Diseases and Self-Management

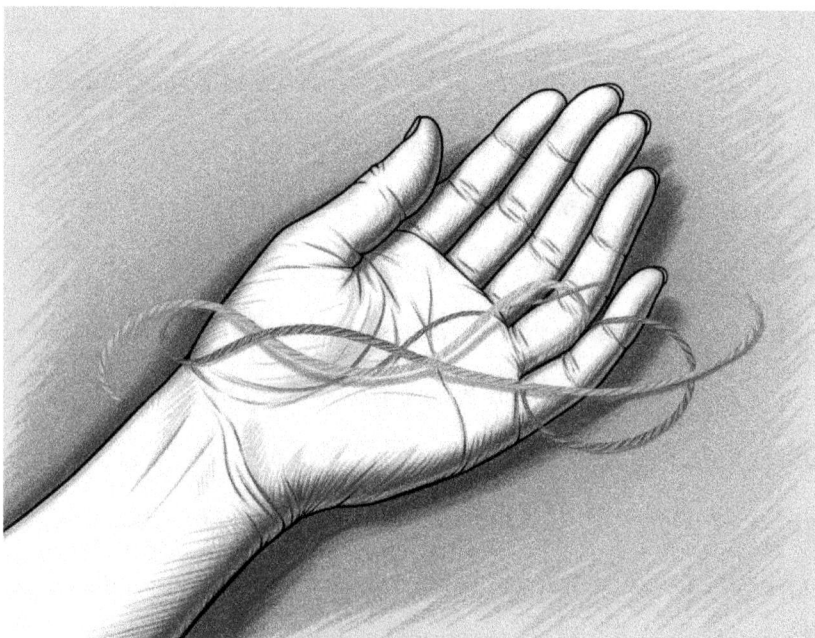

Tip

Building a daily routine is key to managing chronic diseases effectively. Set reminders for medication, schedule regular check-ins with your healthcare team, and use

*simple tracking tools—like a notebook or smartphone app—
to monitor your progress. Small, consistent actions can
make a big difference in controlling symptoms and
improving your quality of life.*

C hronic diseases present a significant challenge in today's
healthcare landscape, impacting millions of people
around the globe. Unlike acute
illnesses, which appear suddenly and resolve quickly, these
conditions persist over time, often requiring ongoing medical
attention and greatly influencing a person's daily life and overall
well-being.

These diseases are alarmingly common. Conditions like
diabetes, **hypertension**, and **musculoskeletal disorders**
rank among the most prevalent. The Centers for Disease Control
and Prevention (CDC) reports that nearly 60% of adults in the
United States have at least one chronic condition, with about
40% managing two or more at the same time. These statistics
highlight the importance of understanding these issues to
develop effective management strategies.

Several key differences distinguish chronic conditions from
acute illnesses. Acute issues, such as influenza or fractures,
typically present clear symptoms that require immediate care
and often resolve with treatment or on their own, allowing
individuals to return to their routines. In contrast, chronic
diseases develop gradually and may not show obvious
symptoms at first. This lack of early warning can delay diagnosis

and treatment, giving the disease time to progress and
potentially lead to more serious health problems.

These conditions often last for years or even a lifetime,
necessitating continuous management to keep symptoms under
control and prevent complications. Because they progress
slowly, individuals might not notice significant changes in their
health until the disease has advanced, which can result in a
gradual decline in quality of life. Everyday activities, work, and
social participation can become increasingly challenging.

Diabetes, **hypertension**, and **musculoskeletal disorders**
are prime examples of chronic diseases that can significantly
affect both individual health and the healthcare system.

- Diabetes, characterized by high blood sugar levels, can
  lead to serious complications like heart disease, kidney
  failure, and nerve damage if not managed effectively.
- Hypertension raises the risk of heart attacks, strokes, and
  other cardiovascular issues.
- Musculoskeletal disorders impact bones, muscles, and
  joints, often causing persistent pain and limited mobility,
  which can make it difficult for individuals to remain
  active and engaged in life.

The effects of chronic conditions extend beyond the individual,
placing a considerable burden on the healthcare system.
Ongoing medical care, medications, and regular check-ups
increase costs and consume significant resources. Managing
these issues often requires a collaborative approach, involving
doctors, nurses, dietitians, and physical therapists, to provide
the comprehensive care and support that individuals need.

A thorough understanding of chronic diseases is essential for effective management and prevention. Recognizing the signs and symptoms enables individuals to seek medical help sooner and make lifestyle changes that can lessen the impact of these conditions. Education and awareness are vital in empowering people to take control of their health and make informed decisions about their care. Consistent self-management each day can lead to better long-term health, improved quality of life, and reduced pressure on the healthcare system.

Daily self-management is a vital aspect of effectively handling chronic conditions, acting as a proactive approach that empowers individuals to take charge of their health. This concept encompasses a series of intentional, consistent actions designed to maintain stability in health status and prevent disease progression. By committing to this practice, individuals can significantly reduce the risk of complications associated with chronic illnesses and enhance their long-term health outcomes.

A key element is the systematic monitoring of symptoms, which involves carefully tracking any changes in one's condition, such as daily blood sugar readings for those with diabetes or regular blood pressure measurements for individuals with hypertension. Keeping a detailed log of these metrics helps identify patterns or triggers that may negatively impact health. This data offers valuable insights for both the individual and healthcare providers, enabling them to tailor treatment plans more effectively.

Following prescribed medication regimens is another crucial part of self-management, as medications are essential for controlling symptoms and preventing disease progression. The effectiveness of these treatments relies on consistent and accurate use, making it important to understand the significance of taking medications as directed, including:

- Timing
- Dosage
- Any specific instructions regarding food interactions or other medications

This level of adherence is necessary for maintaining therapeutic drug levels in the body and achieving the best treatment results.

Lifestyle changes, particularly in nutrition and physical activity, play a significant role in managing chronic diseases. Consuming a well-balanced diet rich in essential nutrients helps regulate body weight, blood sugar, and cholesterol levels, all of which are important for those with chronic conditions. For instance, individuals with diabetes may focus on *carbohydrate counting* and selecting foods with a *low glycemic index* to manage blood sugar levels, while those with hypertension may benefit from a sodium-restricted diet high in potassium to help lower blood pressure.

Regular exercise is equally important, as it supports overall physical health and can alleviate symptoms related to chronic conditions. Consistent physical activity enhances cardiovascular health, boosts insulin sensitivity, and strengthens muscles and bones, which is particularly beneficial for those with musculoskeletal disorders. The goal is to create an enjoyable and sustainable exercise routine, whether that involves walking, swimming, or practicing yoga, and to incorporate it into daily life.

Technology now plays a crucial role in supporting daily self-management, offering a variety of applications and wearable devices that help track health metrics, remind individuals to take medications, and provide personalized feedback on progress. For example, continuous glucose monitors can sync with smartphones to deliver real-time data on blood sugar levels, while fitness trackers can record physical activity and heart rate. These tools simplify the management of chronic conditions and foster accountability and motivation.

Moreover, technology enhances communication with healthcare providers, as many applications allow users to share health data directly with their physicians. This direct exchange of information leads to more informed discussions during appointments, resulting in more personalized care and timely adjustments to treatment plans, which can ultimately improve health outcomes.

Managing diabetes requires a strong focus on self-care to maintain health and prevent complications. One of the most important habits is checking blood glucose levels regularly, ideally at least four times a day. This routine helps individuals understand how their bodies respond to different foods, activities, and medications. Keeping a detailed log of readings, along with the time and what was eaten, makes it easier to identify trends and make informed choices about diet and insulin. Taking these steps helps keep blood sugar within target

ranges and reduces the risk of long-term issues like **diabetic
neuropathy** or **heart disease**.

Diet plays a major role in managing diabetes. A balanced
approach that includes:

- Whole grains
- Lean proteins
- A variety of non-starchy vegetables

helps stabilize blood sugar. Counting carbohydrates at each
meal is a practical way to manage intake and avoid spikes in
glucose. Choosing foods with a low *glycemic index*, such as
legumes and whole fruits, also supports stable levels. Planning
meals ahead of time, preparing healthy snacks, and being
mindful of portion sizes and meal timing all contribute to
preventing swings.

Physical activity is another key part of diabetes self-care.
Exercise enhances **insulin sensitivity**, allowing the body to
use glucose more efficiently. Activities like brisk walking,
cycling, or swimming can easily fit into daily life, and setting
realistic goals—such as 150 minutes of moderate aerobic
exercise each week—makes it easier to maintain a routine.
Incorporating strength training twice a week builds muscle
mass, which further aids in regulating glucose.

People managing hypertension benefit from regular blood
pressure checks. Tracking readings at the same time each day
reveals how lifestyle factors, including diet and stress, influence
blood pressure. This information helps guide adjustments to

keep it in a healthy range, usually below **130/80 mmHg**. Reducing sodium intake is a significant dietary change that can have a big impact. Opting for fresh, unprocessed foods and using herbs and spices instead of salt makes this transition smoother.

Maintaining a healthy weight is also important for controlling hypertension. Extra weight puts more strain on the heart and blood vessels, raising blood pressure. Eating a diet rich in fruits, vegetables, and whole grains, along with regular exercise, supports weight management. Simple changes, like taking the stairs or adding short walks throughout the day, can lead to gradual weight loss and improved heart health.

For those with musculoskeletal issues, physical therapy can help manage pain and maintain mobility. A licensed physical therapist can create a personalized exercise plan that targets problem areas, focusing on building strength and flexibility. Doing these exercises at home makes it easier to incorporate them into daily routines, and sticking with the program leads to better function and less pain.

Adjusting work and home environments to be more ergonomic can also alleviate discomfort from musculoskeletal disorders. Setting up workstations to promote good posture and reduce strain helps prevent symptoms from worsening. Simple changes, like ensuring chairs are the right height or using a footrest, can significantly enhance comfort.

Exercises that focus on mobility and pain relief are important for individuals with musculoskeletal concerns. Stretching improves flexibility, and low-impact activities like swimming or tai chi boost fitness without stressing the joints. Finding enjoyable activities that can be done regularly is key to staying committed to an exercise routine.

Managing chronic diseases involves not just physical adjustments but also a significant psychological and motivational commitment. Self-management can often feel daunting due to the ongoing dedication it requires, and one of the biggest hurdles is keeping motivation alive over time. The daily tasks of monitoring health metrics, sticking to medication schedules, and making lifestyle changes can feel heavy, sometimes leading to burnout or complacency. Setting realistic and achievable goals can make this journey more manageable. By breaking down larger objectives into smaller, measurable tasks, you can reduce feelings of intimidation and make progress feel more rewarding. For instance, rather than aiming to lose a large amount of weight all at once, consider setting a target of losing **1-2 pounds** per week or adding an extra **10 minutes** of physical activity to your daily routine.

Tracking your progress is essential for sustaining motivation. Using a journal or digital tools to record achievements, no matter how small, fosters a sense of accomplishment and reinforces positive habits. This method not only highlights improvements but also reveals areas that may need a bit more focus. Celebrating small wins, like reaching a new exercise milestone or keeping blood sugar levels within target ranges for a week, can lift your spirits and encourage continued effort.

A strong support network is vital for maintaining motivation and accountability. Involving healthcare professionals, family, and friends provides the encouragement needed to stay on track. Healthcare providers can offer expert advice and adjust treatment plans to ensure management strategies remain effective. Loved ones can provide emotional support and practical assistance, such as joining you for exercise or helping with meal preparation. Connecting with others who are facing similar health challenges, whether through support groups or online communities, fosters a sense of camaraderie and offers additional motivation through shared experiences and strategies.

Education and self-awareness empower individuals to take charge of their health. Gaining a clear understanding of your condition and the effects of different management strategies can make the process less confusing and diminish feelings of helplessness. Attending workshops, reading current literature, or participating in educational programs builds knowledge and confidence, enabling you to make informed choices about your care and advocate for yourself in healthcare settings.

Recognizing personal triggers and stressors that interfere with self-management is a crucial aspect of self-awareness. Identifying these factors allows you to develop coping strategies and make necessary adjustments to your daily routine. For example, if stress leads to unhealthy eating, practicing stress-reduction techniques like *mindfulness meditation* or *deep-breathing exercises* can help counteract this tendency. Being attentive to your emotional and physical responses also makes it easier to anticipate challenges and prepare for them in advance.

Chronic Diseases and the Power of Daily Habits

Chronic diseases pose a significant challenge in today's healthcare landscape, marked by their long-lasting nature and persistent symptoms. Unlike acute illnesses that strike suddenly and resolve quickly, these conditions develop gradually and require ongoing management. This slow progression often leads to subtle symptoms that can be easily overlooked, potentially delaying diagnosis and treatment. Consequently, individuals may find their quality of life gradually declining, making everyday tasks increasingly challenging.

Diabetes, hypertension, and musculoskeletal disorders are among the most common chronic conditions, each presenting unique challenges for patients and the healthcare system. **Diabetes** is characterized by the body's difficulty in regulating blood sugar, which can result in serious complications such as heart disease, kidney failure, and nerve damage if not managed effectively. **Hypertension**, or high blood pressure, significantly heightens the risk of heart attacks and strokes. **Musculoskeletal disorders** often lead to persistent pain and restricted movement, making it tougher for individuals to remain active and engage in daily activities.

These conditions impact not only those diagnosed but also place a considerable strain on the healthcare system. Ongoing medical appointments, prescription medications, and regular check-ups can drive up costs and consume valuable resources. Effective management typically requires a collaborative approach, with doctors, nurses, dietitians, and physical therapists working together to provide comprehensive care and support.

Consistent self-management is essential for controlling chronic diseases and preventing complications. This approach involves:

- Following prescribed medications as directed
- Making lifestyle adjustments
- Regularly monitoring health

For instance, individuals with diabetes should frequently check their blood sugar, stick to their medication schedule, and maintain a balanced diet to keep their condition in check. Those with hypertension benefit from regular blood pressure monitoring, reducing salt intake, and staying physically active to maintain a healthy range.

A proactive mindset and informed decision-making empower individuals to successfully integrate these habits into their daily routines. Education and self-awareness are vital in enabling effective health management. When people understand their condition and the impact of various management strategies, they can make informed choices about their care and advocate for themselves in healthcare settings.

New technology enhances daily self-management by providing apps and wearable devices that track health data, remind users to take medications, and offer personalized feedback. For example, *continuous glucose monitors* can sync with smartphones to provide real-time blood sugar updates, while

fitness trackers can log activity levels and heart rate, making it
easier to manage chronic conditions and stay motivated.

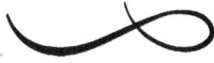

Chapter 2: Types, Causes, and Symptoms of Diabetes

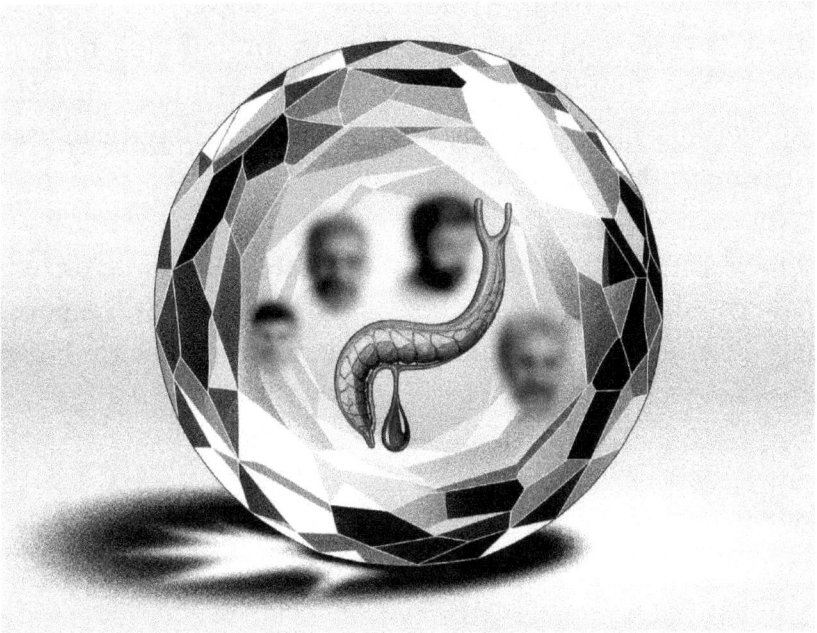

D iabetes is a multifaceted condition that comes in various forms, each with unique characteristics and management needs. Grasping these differences is essential for effectively managing the disease and preventing complications. The three primary types—Type 1, Type 2, and Gestational Diabetes—each present specific challenges and require tailored management strategies.

Type 1 diabetes is an autoimmune disorder where the immune system mistakenly attacks the insulin-producing beta cells in the pancreas, resulting in a complete lack of insulin, a hormone vital for regulating blood glucose levels. Typically diagnosed in childhood or early adulthood, this type necessitates lifelong insulin therapy to maintain blood sugar control. Individuals need to monitor their glucose levels regularly, often using continuous glucose monitors or fingerstick tests, and administer insulin through injections or a pump. This routine is crucial for preventing immediate complications like diabetic ketoacidosis and long-term issues such as neuropathy and retinopathy.

The most prevalent form, **Type 2 diabetes**, is characterized by insulin resistance, where the body's cells become less responsive to the hormone. This type is often associated with lifestyle factors such as:

- High-calorie diets
- Insufficient physical activity
- Obesity

Management usually begins with lifestyle modifications, including dietary changes to lower refined carbohydrates and boost fiber intake, along with regular exercise. As the condition progresses, medication or insulin therapy may be required. The gradual onset of Type 2 diabetes can make symptoms less apparent, so early detection and intervention are crucial for avoiding complications like heart disease and kidney failure.

Gestational diabetes arises during pregnancy when hormonal changes hinder insulin's effectiveness, leading to elevated blood sugar levels. While this type typically resolves after childbirth, it increases the risk of developing Type 2 diabetes later for both mother and child. Routine prenatal screenings, such as the oral glucose tolerance test, are essential for early detection. Management often involves dietary adjustments and, in some cases, insulin therapy to maintain stable glucose levels throughout pregnancy.

Both genetic and environmental factors contribute to the development of diabetes. Type 1 has a strong genetic component, but environmental triggers, such as certain viral infections, can initiate the autoimmune response. For Type 2, genetics play a role, but lifestyle choices—like eating habits and activity levels—are significant contributors. High-calorie diets, inactivity, and obesity greatly elevate risk, and metabolic syndrome—a cluster of conditions including high blood pressure, abnormal cholesterol, and central obesity—further increases the likelihood of developing the disease. In gestational diabetes, pregnancy hormones can disrupt insulin function, making careful monitoring and management essential to safeguard both mother and baby.

Recognizing symptoms early is vital for timely diagnosis and effective treatment. **Type 1 diabetes** often presents with clear signs such as:

- Frequent urination
- Intense thirst
- Unexplained weight loss

- Fatigue
- Blurred vision

Symptoms of **Type 2** tend to be more subtle, including:

- Increased thirst
- Frequent urination
- Heightened hunger
- Fatigue
- Slow-healing wounds

Gestational diabetes may not produce noticeable symptoms and is frequently detected through routine prenatal tests. Early detection and diagnosis are crucial for preventing complications and initiating appropriate treatment.

Being attentive to symptoms and seeking medical advice promptly are important steps in recognizing and managing diabetes. Regular check-ups and screenings are especially important for individuals with risk factors like a family history of the condition or obesity. Self-monitoring, such as using glucometers to track blood sugar levels and maintaining a symptom diary, can help identify patterns and triggers. Healthcare professionals play a key role in confirming diagnoses and developing personalized management plans, which may include dietary guidance, exercise recommendations, and medication adjustments.

Tip

If you have a family history of diabetes or notice symptoms like increased thirst or fatigue, schedule a screening with your healthcare provider. Early detection can make a significant difference in managing diabetes and preventing complications. Keep a simple symptom diary and track your blood sugar if possible—these small steps can empower you to take control of your health, even with a busy lifestyle.

Types, Causes, and Early Signs of Diabetes

A clear understanding of the physiological mechanisms behind diabetes is essential for effective management and prevention strategies. **Type 1 diabetes** occurs when the immune system mistakenly targets and destroys the insulin-producing beta cells in the pancreas, leading to a complete lack of insulin, a hormone necessary for cells to absorb glucose and produce energy. Without it, glucose builds up in the bloodstream, causing **hyperglycemia**. Individuals with Type 1 diabetes rely on **insulin therapy** to mimic the natural secretion patterns of a healthy pancreas. This approach requires frequent blood glucose monitoring, often several times a day, and the use of subcutaneous injections or insulin pumps to maintain optimal glycemic control and reduce the risk of complications such as **diabetic ketoacidosis**.

Type 2 diabetes, on the other hand, is primarily characterized by **insulin resistance**, where the body's cells respond less effectively to this hormone. Initially, the pancreas compensates by producing more insulin, but this response eventually fails, resulting in persistent hyperglycemia. This form of diabetes is often linked to lifestyle factors such as:

- Poor diet
- Lack of physical activity
- Obesity

However, targeted lifestyle changes can slow or even reverse the progression of insulin resistance. A balanced diet focused on whole grains, lean proteins, and healthy fats, combined with regular physical activity—at least 150 minutes of moderate-intensity exercise per week—can significantly improve insulin sensitivity and help manage the condition.

Gestational diabetes develops during pregnancy when hormones from the placenta interfere with insulin's effectiveness, causing resistance. Careful monitoring of blood glucose levels is necessary to protect both the mother and the developing fetus. Although this condition usually resolves after childbirth, it increases the risk of developing Type 2 diabetes later in life for both mother and child. Regular prenatal screenings, such as glucose tolerance tests, along with a nutritious diet and physical activity during pregnancy, play a vital role in management.

Recognizing early warning signs allows for timely intervention. **Prediabetes**, which often precedes Type 2 diabetes, is marked by elevated fasting glucose levels or A1C results between 5.7% and 6.4%. These numbers indicate the body is struggling to maintain normal blood sugar levels. Being aware of personal risk factors—such as age, family history, ethnicity, and lifestyle choices—enables individuals to take proactive steps to lower their risk. Preventive strategies include:

- Reaching and maintaining a healthy weight
- Staying physically active
- Following a balanced diet that limits processed sugars and saturated fats

Stress management and sufficient sleep are also important for metabolic health. Chronic stress and lack of sleep can negatively impact insulin sensitivity and glycemic control. Stress-reduction techniques like *yoga, mindfulness meditation*, or *deep breathing exercises*, along with getting 7-9 hours of quality sleep each night, can enhance overall well-being and metabolic function.

Working closely with healthcare providers helps create a comprehensive management plan. Regular monitoring of blood glucose, blood pressure, and lipid profiles is necessary to track progress and make informed treatment adjustments. Setting realistic health goals and building a supportive environment are crucial for maintaining long-term diabetes management. Support from family and friends, participation in education programs, and the use of digital health tools such as mobile apps and wearable devices can help track health metrics and sustain motivation.

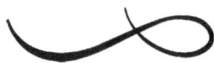

Chapter 3: Key Facts and Early Signs of Hypertension

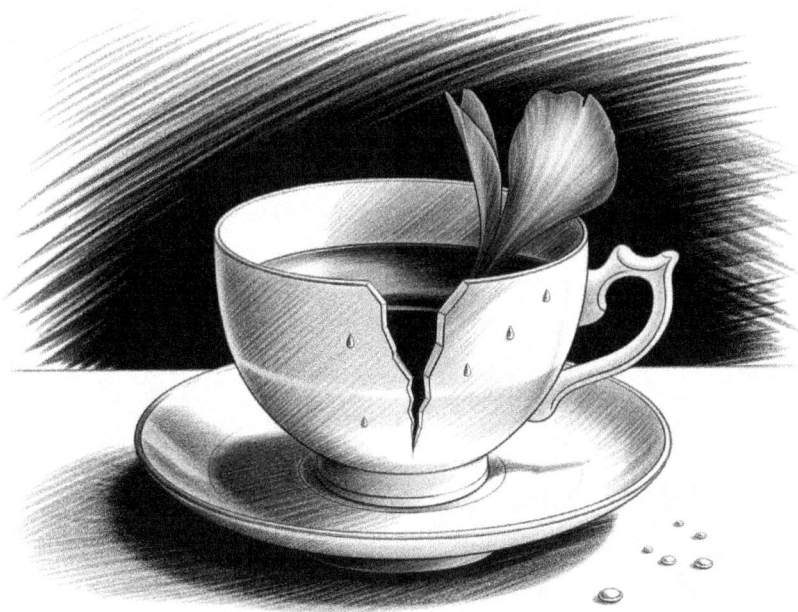

Hypertension, often known as **high blood pressure**, is a chronic medical condition where blood consistently exerts elevated pressure against the arterial walls. Diagnosis hinges on two key measurements: **systolic** and **diastolic pressure**. The systolic value, which is the higher number, measures the pressure in the arteries during the heart's contraction, while the diastolic value reflects the pressure during the relaxation phase between heartbeats. A typical healthy reading is around 120/80 mmHg, and the condition is diagnosed when these numbers consistently exceed 130/80 mmHg.

There are two main types of hypertension:

- **Primary hypertension**, also referred to as *essential hypertension*, is the most common form and typically develops gradually over several years. Factors such as genetics, including family history, and lifestyle choices like diet and physical activity play a significant role.
- **Secondary hypertension** arises from identifiable underlying conditions, such as kidney disease, endocrine disorders like *hyperthyroidism*, or side effects from certain medications, including hormonal contraceptives and decongestants. Identifying the specific type is crucial for selecting the most effective management and treatment strategies.

Several risk factors can increase the likelihood of developing this condition. Age is a major factor, with the risk rising as people get older. A family history of hypertension also elevates the risk. Lifestyle choices are important as well; obesity, lack of physical activity, and a diet high in sodium and low in potassium contribute to higher blood pressure. Excessive alcohol consumption and chronic stress also play a role, so recognizing and addressing these factors is vital for prevention and early intervention.

Often referred to as the "silent killer," hypertension can exist without noticeable symptoms. Some individuals may experience warning signs such as:

- Frequent headaches
- Dizziness
- Shortness of breath
- Nosebleeds

These symptoms should not be overlooked, as they can indicate dangerously high blood pressure. Regular checks are essential for early detection and can help prevent complications like cardiovascular disease, stroke, and kidney damage.

Effectively managing the condition usually requires both lifestyle changes and, when necessary, medication. Key dietary changes include:

- Reducing sodium intake, as high salt consumption is linked to increased blood pressure.
- Eating a balanced diet rich in fruits, vegetables, whole grains, and lean proteins to support healthy levels.
- Engaging in regular physical activity, such as brisk walking, cycling, or swimming, with at least 150 minutes of moderate-intensity exercise recommended each week.

Cutting back on alcohol and avoiding tobacco are important steps for control. Alcohol can raise blood pressure, and smoking damages blood vessels, worsening the condition. Stress management techniques like meditation, yoga, and deep-breathing exercises can help control blood pressure by promoting relaxation and reducing stress.

Collaborating closely with healthcare providers is essential for anyone diagnosed with hypertension. A personalized management plan may include medication for those whose levels remain high. Common medications include:

- Diuretics
- ACE inhibitors
- Beta-blockers

All are aimed at lowering blood pressure. Adhering to the prescribed treatment plan and attending regular follow-up appointments are necessary for tracking progress and making any needed adjustments.

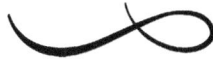

Chapter 4: Understanding Musculoskeletal Disorders

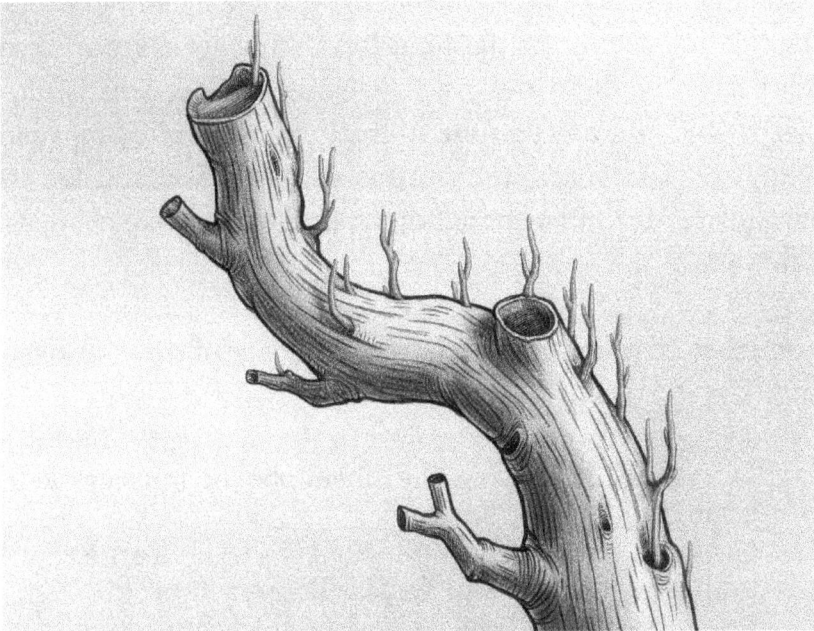

Musculoskeletal disorders include a range of conditions that affect the body's structural framework, such as bones, muscles, joints, and connective tissues. Common examples are **osteoarthritis**, **rheumatoid arthritis**, **osteoporosis**, and **lower back pain**. Each of these conditions affects the musculoskeletal system in its own way, often leading to symptoms like localized pain, joint stiffness, inflammation, and reduced mobility.

Osteoarthritis is the most common type of arthritis, occurring when cartilage—the protective tissue at the ends of bones—gradually breaks down. This wear and tear causes bones to rub against each other, resulting in significant pain and swelling in the affected joints. On the other hand, **rheumatoid arthritis** is an autoimmune disorder where the immune system mistakenly attacks the synovial membrane, leading to joint inflammation and potential long-term damage. **Osteoporosis** is characterized by a decrease in bone density, which makes bones fragile and more prone to fractures, especially in weight-bearing areas. **Lower back pain** is also prevalent and can stem from muscle strain, herniated discs, or degenerative changes in the lumbar spine.

Several factors contribute to the development of these disorders:

- Aging, as the body's ability to repair tissues diminishes over time, increasing the likelihood of musculoskeletal issues.
- Genetics, with some individuals being more susceptible to these conditions due to hereditary factors.
- Previous injuries, which may lead to chronic pain.
- Repetitive strain from certain jobs, which can accelerate wear and tear on the musculoskeletal system.
- A sedentary lifestyle, which can result in muscle weakness and joint stiffness, further raising the risk of these disorders.

These conditions can greatly affect daily life, making routine activities more challenging. Pain and stiffness can complicate basic movements like walking or climbing stairs. A limited range of motion may hinder reaching overhead or bending down, while chronic pain often leads to persistent fatigue, which can lower energy levels and overall quality of life.

Managing symptoms effectively relies on evidence-based strategies. Regular low-impact exercise, such as *swimming* or *yoga*, helps maintain joint flexibility and muscle strength without putting excessive stress on the body. A balanced diet rich in calcium and vitamin D supports bone health, and using ergonomic tools and supportive footwear can help reduce strain on joints and muscles.

Physical therapy and occupational therapy play vital roles in improving function and alleviating pain. Physical therapists design personalized exercise programs to enhance strength and flexibility, while occupational therapists recommend modifications to daily routines and environments to minimize strain and improve comfort.

Open communication with healthcare professionals is crucial for creating treatment plans tailored to individual needs. These plans may include medications like **nonsteroidal anti-inflammatory drugs (NSAIDs)** or **corticosteroids** to help manage pain and inflammation. Incorporating stretching routines, maintaining good posture, and using assistive devices can also make daily activities easier and more comfortable.

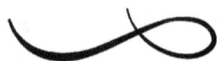

Chapter 5: Lifestyle Choices for Chronic Disease Control

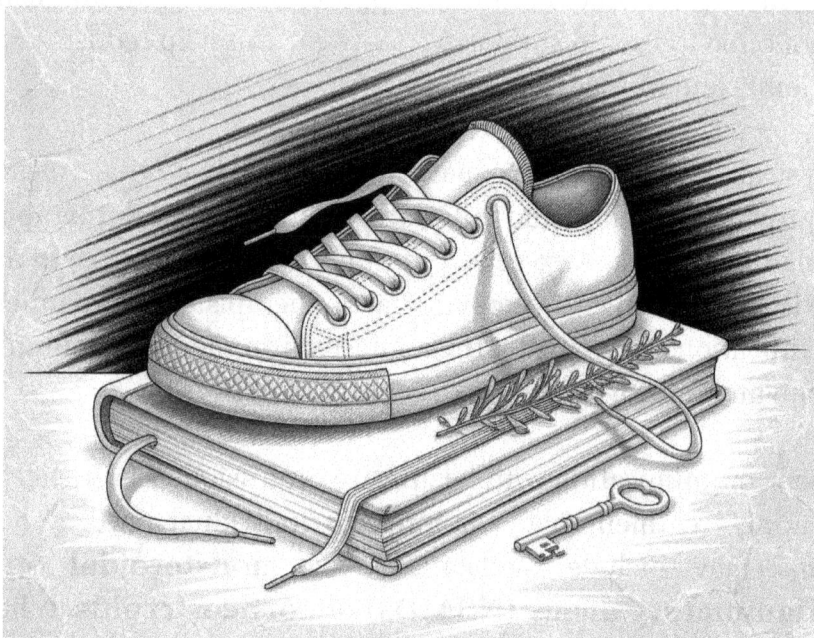

Tip

If you're short on time or resources, focus on small, sustainable changes. Prepping healthy snacks in advance, taking short walks during breaks, and setting a regular bedtime can make a big difference. Consistency, not perfection, is key—small steps add up to better control of chronic conditions.

L ifestyle choices play a vital role in managing chronic diseases, especially diabetes, hypertension, and musculoskeletal disorders. By focusing on key areas like diet, physical activity, and sleep, individuals can make a significant impact on their health outcomes. These elements are essential for both preventing and managing chronic conditions, serving as important complements to medical treatments.

Diet is a fundamental factor in controlling these diseases. Embracing a balanced and nutritious eating plan tailored to individual health needs can lead to meaningful improvements. It's important to limit processed foods, refined sugars, and sodium, as these often contain unhealthy fats and additives that can worsen conditions like hypertension and diabetes. Opting for whole grains, lean proteins, fruits, vegetables, and healthy fats is a great choice. Whole grains such as brown rice and quinoa provide essential nutrients and dietary fiber, which help stabilize blood sugar and support heart health. Lean proteins like chicken, fish, and legumes are crucial for muscle maintenance and repair, especially for those with musculoskeletal disorders. Fruits and vegetables offer a wide array of vitamins, minerals, and antioxidants that help reduce inflammation and promote overall well-being. Healthy fats from sources like avocados, nuts, and olive oil are beneficial for heart health and can assist with weight management.

Practical strategies for meal planning and preparation can make these dietary changes easier to implement. Consider the following strategies:

- Practice portion control, such as using smaller plates, to help reduce portion sizes while still keeping meals satisfying.
- Eat mindfully—taking the time to savor each bite—to enhance the dining experience and help prevent overeating.
- Plan meals in advance and prep ingredients to save time and lessen the temptation to reach for unhealthy convenience foods.

Physical activity is another crucial element in managing chronic diseases. Different types of exercise provide unique benefits for each condition. Aerobic exercises like walking, cycling, and swimming are particularly effective for improving cardiovascular health and insulin sensitivity. These activities help lower blood pressure and enhance circulation, which is beneficial for those managing hypertension and diabetes. Strength training, including weight lifting and resistance exercises, builds and maintains muscle mass, supporting the musculoskeletal system and aiding in weight control. Flexibility exercises such as yoga and stretching improve joint mobility and reduce the risk of injury, which is especially important for individuals with musculoskeletal issues.

Setting realistic fitness goals can help maintain motivation and track progress. Consider the following steps:

- Start with small, achievable targets—like a daily 10-minute walk.
- Gradually increase duration and intensity as fitness improves.
- Keep a fitness journal or use a mobile app to log workouts, fostering a sense of accomplishment and revealing patterns or areas that may need attention.

Staying motivated can be challenging at times, but choosing enjoyable activities and weaving them into daily routines can make exercise more appealing. Joining a class or working out with a partner can also provide social support and enhance accountability.

Sleep is a vital foundation for managing chronic diseases and is essential for maintaining overall health and well-being. Quality rest is crucial for hormone regulation, which significantly influences conditions like diabetes, hypertension, and musculoskeletal pain. During this restorative time, the body effectively regulates **insulin** and **cortisol** levels, both of which are key for managing blood sugar and stress. Getting enough sleep also helps reduce inflammation—a common contributor to many chronic conditions—by modulating inflammatory markers such as *C-reactive protein (CRP)* and *interleukin-6 (IL-6)*.

To reap the benefits of sleep, it's important to create a sleep-friendly environment and establish a consistent routine. Consider the following tips:

- Go to bed and wake up at the same time each day to regulate your body's circadian rhythm.

- Choose a supportive mattress and pillows that suit your preferred sleep positions.
- Keep the room dark and quiet, aiming for a cool temperature, ideally between 60-67°F.
- Use blackout curtains or a sleep mask to block out light.
- Minimize disruptive sounds with earplugs or a white noise machine.

It's also crucial to avoid stimulants before bedtime. **Caffeine**, found in coffee, tea, and many sodas, can interfere with your ability to fall and stay asleep, with effects lasting up to six hours after consumption. Limiting caffeine intake after 2 PM is a smart move. Additionally, electronic devices like smartphones, tablets, and computers emit blue light, which can suppress **melatonin** production—a hormone that promotes sleep. Reducing screen time at least one hour before bed allows melatonin levels to rise naturally, which can improve sleep quality.

Common sleep disorders, such as sleep apnea and insomnia, can significantly impact chronic disease management. **Sleep apnea**, characterized by repeated interruptions in breathing during sleep, can elevate blood pressure and worsen cardiovascular issues, increasing the risk of heart attack and stroke. **Insomnia,** or difficulty falling or staying asleep, leads to chronic fatigue and impaired cognitive function, affecting daily activities and overall health. If you experience persistent disturbances, seeking professional advice is important, as healthcare providers can offer guidance and potential treatments, such as **continuous positive airway pressure (CPAP)** therapy for sleep apnea or **cognitive behavioral**

therapy for insomnia. Clinical studies have shown that these treatments can lead to improved outcomes.

Incorporating stress management and relaxation techniques into your daily routine can further enhance sleep quality. Practices like meditation, deep breathing exercises, and progressive muscle relaxation help calm the mind and prepare the body for rest. Consider these techniques:

- **Meditation**: Focus your attention on the breath or a specific mantra to achieve relaxation and mindfulness, which can lower cortisol levels.
- **Deep breathing exercises**: Involve slow, deliberate breaths to activate the parasympathetic nervous system, reduce stress, and promote calm.
- **Progressive muscle relaxation**: Systematically tense and then relax each muscle group, releasing physical tension and encouraging relaxation.

Diet, exercise, and sleep are closely interconnected, and improvements in one area often lead to positive changes in the others, supporting a holistic approach to chronic disease management. For instance, regular physical activity—aiming for at least 150 minutes of moderate aerobic exercise per week—can enhance sleep quality by reducing stress and promoting relaxation. A balanced diet rich in nutrients such as *omega-3 fatty acids, fiber*, and *antioxidants* supports overall health and can boost energy levels, making it easier to stay active and maintain a consistent sleep schedule.

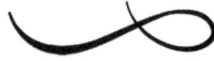

Chapter 6: Building a Positive, Supportive Mindset

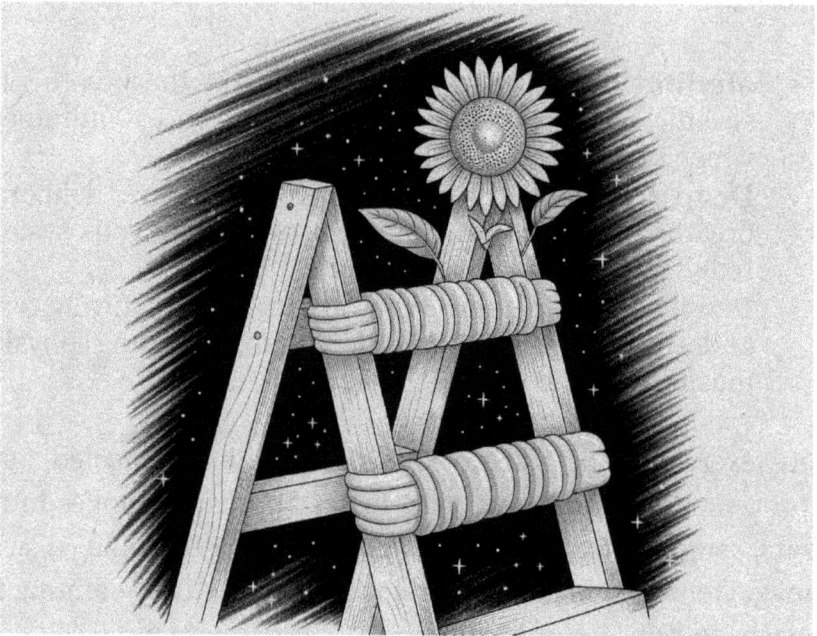

Tip

Building a positive mindset doesn't require big changes—start small. Try writing down one thing you're grateful for each day or take a few minutes to practice mindful breathing. These simple habits can boost your motivation, help you manage stress, and make it easier to stick to your health goals, even on busy days. Remember, progress is about consistency, not perfection. Celebrate each small step forward.

A positive mindset is the cornerstone of effective self-management for chronic diseases. When individuals cultivate a supportive mental framework, they enhance their motivation, improve adherence to treatment plans, and elevate their overall quality of life. Approaching health with optimism and resilience encourages behaviors that promote well-being and effectively manage their conditions.

Self-awareness is the first step toward fostering a positive outlook. This journey involves recognizing and understanding one's thoughts, emotions, and behaviors in detail. By becoming more aware of these internal processes, individuals can identify negative thought patterns that may impede their progress. Thoughts like **"I can't do this"** or **"It's too hard"** can create significant barriers to effective self-management. Once these thoughts are acknowledged, it becomes possible to challenge and reframe them into more constructive alternatives.

Cognitive-behavioral techniques provide practical tools for transforming negative thoughts into more helpful ones. This approach focuses on identifying irrational or unhelpful thoughts and replacing them with balanced, realistic perspectives. For example, instead of thinking, *"I'll never be able to manage my condition,"* a person might say, *"Managing my condition is challenging, but I can take small, measurable steps each day to improve my health."* This shift can significantly boost motivation and adherence to treatment plans.

Self-compassion and acceptance are vital in managing chronic conditions. Practicing patience and forgiveness with oneself is essential while navigating the complexities of living with a chronic disease. Self-compassion means treating oneself with the same kindness and understanding one would offer a friend, recognizing that setbacks are a natural part of the journey rather than a sign of personal failure. Acceptance involves acknowledging the reality of one's condition without judgment, allowing individuals to focus on what they can control and make proactive choices to enhance their health.

Practical exercises can help build resilience and reinforce a positive mindset. Consider the following activities:

- Keeping a gratitude journal: Regularly noting specific things to be thankful for shifts attention from perceived deficiencies to the abundance present in life, enhancing emotional well-being and encouraging a more optimistic outlook.
- Setting achievable personal goals: Breaking down larger objectives into smaller, manageable steps provides individuals with a sense of accomplishment and progress. Celebrating small victories, no matter how minor, reinforces positive behavior and boosts motivation. For instance, if the goal is to incorporate more physical activity into daily life, acknowledging the completion of a 10-minute walk can inspire continued efforts toward that success.

Mindfulness practices are excellent for reducing stress and improving emotional well-being. This involves paying attention to the present moment without judgment. Such practices increase awareness of thoughts and feelings, making it easier to respond to stressors with calm and clarity. Mindfulness meditation is a simple yet powerful technique that can easily fit into daily routines. To start, find a quiet space, sit comfortably, close your eyes, and focus on your breath, noticing the sensation of air entering and leaving your body. When the mind wanders, gently bring your attention back to the breath. Begin with just a few minutes each day and gradually increase the duration as you become more comfortable with the practice.

Mindful breathing is another technique that integrates seamlessly into daily life. This method involves taking slow, deep breaths and focusing on the rhythm of inhalation and exhalation. It can be especially helpful during moments of stress or anxiety, as it activates the body's relaxation response and promotes calm. To practice mindful breathing, inhale deeply through the nose, hold the breath briefly, and then exhale slowly through the mouth. Repeat this process several times, allowing your body to relax with each breath.

A supportive network is essential for fostering a positive mindset and enhancing self-management. Family, friends, and peer groups provide crucial emotional support, encouragement, and practical help tailored to your unique needs. Open communication is the cornerstone of these relationships. By sharing specific experiences and discussing particular challenges, you help others understand and empathize, which is vital for building strong connections.

To cultivate and strengthen your support system, reach out to loved ones, clearly express your needs, and discuss specific aspects of your situation. This openness allows them to grasp what you're experiencing and offer the right kind of assistance. Encouraging questions and sharing thoughts create a two-way conversation that enriches your relationship. Involving family and friends in your self-management activities, such as:

- Inviting them for a walk
- Asking for help with meal preparation
- Sharing experiences during activities

not only provides practical support but also deepens your bond through shared experiences.

Peer groups, whether in-person or online, offer valuable opportunities to connect with others who are facing similar challenges. These communities enable you to share insights, exchange practical tips, and receive encouragement from those who truly understand your situation. Online forums and social media groups are particularly beneficial for those with busy schedules, as they provide flexibility and easy access. When you join these groups, take an active role by sharing your experiences and supporting others. This mutual exchange fosters a sense of belonging and strengthens the community.

Healthcare professionals also play a vital role in providing emotional support and guidance. To communicate your needs and concerns effectively during medical appointments, prepare in advance by jotting down specific questions and describing any symptoms or challenges you're facing. Being honest and open about your feelings and any difficulties in managing your condition allows providers to offer advice and support that aligns with your situation. If you believe that referrals to mental health professionals or support groups could be beneficial, don't hesitate to ask for them to enhance your overall well-being.

Personal relationships flourish through **active listening**, **empathy**, and **gratitude**. Active listening means giving your full attention to what the other person is saying, without interrupting or planning your response while they speak. This demonstrates respect and understanding, which can deepen your connection. *Empathy* involves seeing things from the other person's perspective and recognizing their feelings. Expressing empathy validates their emotions and helps create a supportive environment. Showing gratitude, whether through words or small gestures, encourages positive interactions and strengthens your relationships. A simple thank-you note or a heartfelt conversation can significantly express appreciation for the support you receive.

EXERCISE 1. MEAL PLANNING FOR BALANCED BLOOD SUGAR

Objective

Create a meal plan that maintains balanced blood sugar levels throughout the day, supporting effective self-management of diabetes.

Step-by-step instructions

- Identify your daily caloric needs based on your age, weight, activity level, and health goals. Consult with a healthcare provider if needed.

- Divide your daily caloric intake into three main meals and two snacks. Aim for consistent meal times to stabilize blood sugar levels.

- For each meal, include a balance of macronutrients:
- Carbohydrates: Choose complex carbs like whole grains, legumes, and vegetables. Limit simple sugars.
- Proteins: Incorporate lean proteins such as chicken, fish, tofu, or beans.
- Fats: Opt for healthy fats like avocados, nuts, and olive oil.

- Use the plate method for portion control:
- Fill half your plate with non-starchy vegetables.
- One-quarter with lean protein.
- One-quarter with whole grains or starchy vegetables.

- Monitor portion sizes using measuring cups or a food scale to ensure accuracy.

- Plan snacks that include protein and fiber to prevent blood sugar spikes, such as a small apple with almond butter or Greek yogurt with berries.

- Stay hydrated by drinking water throughout the day. Limit sugary drinks and alcohol.

- Prepare meals in advance to avoid last-minute unhealthy choices. Batch cook and store meals in portioned containers.

- Keep a food diary to track what you eat and how it affects your blood sugar levels. Adjust your plan as needed based on these observations.

Common pitfalls

- Skipping meals, which can lead to blood sugar fluctuations.
- Over-relying on processed foods that may contain hidden sugars and unhealthy fats.
- Ignoring portion sizes, leading to excessive calorie intake.

Progress tracking

- Regularly check your blood sugar levels before and after meals to assess the effectiveness of your meal plan.
- Review your food diary weekly to identify patterns and make necessary adjustments.
- Set specific, achievable goals for meal planning and track your progress over time.

MANAGING CHRONIC DISEASES: A PRACTICAL GUIDE TO DAILY CONTROL OF
DIABETES, HYPERTENSION, AND MUSCULOSKELETAL ISSUES

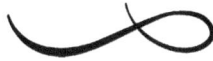

Chapter 7: Physical Activity for Beginners

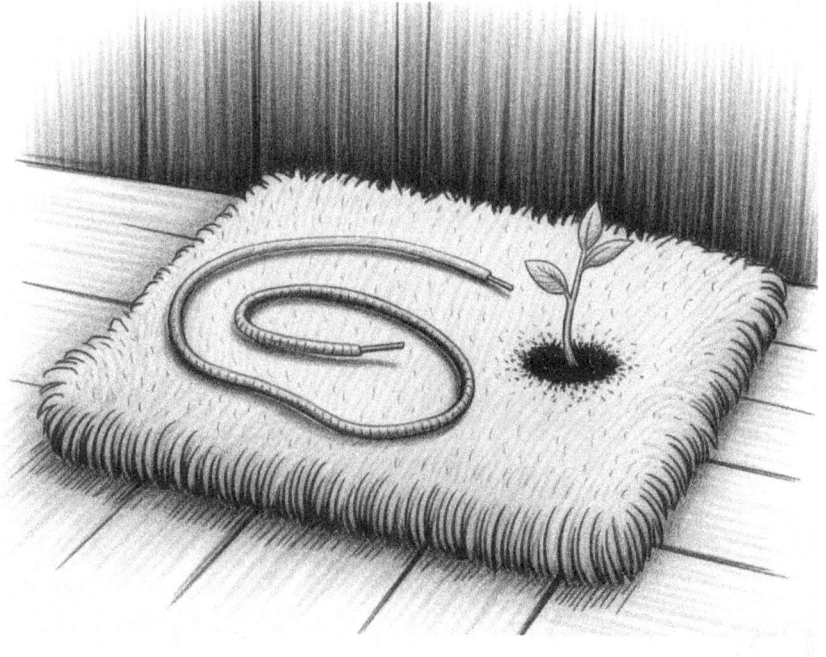

EXERCISE 2. WALKING FOR BEGINNERS

Objective

Introduce a simple walking routine to improve cardiovascular health, manage weight, and enhance overall well-being.

Step-by-step instructions

- Choose a safe, flat route for your walk, such as a local park or neighborhood sidewalk. Aim for a path that is well-lit and free of obstacles.

- Wear comfortable, supportive shoes to prevent injury and ensure proper foot alignment.

- Begin with a 5-minute warm-up by walking at a slow, relaxed pace to gradually increase your heart rate.

- Increase your pace to a brisk walk, aiming for a speed where you can still hold a conversation but feel slightly out of breath. Maintain this pace for 10-15 minutes.

- Focus on maintaining good posture: keep your head up, shoulders relaxed, and arms swinging naturally at your sides.

- Cool down with a 5-minute slow walk to gradually lower your heart rate.

- Stretch your major muscle groups, including calves, thighs, and lower back, to prevent stiffness and improve flexibility.

- Gradually increase your walking duration by 5 minutes each week until you reach a total of 30 minutes per session.

- Aim to walk at least 5 days a week for optimal health benefits.

Common pitfalls

- Walking too fast too soon, which can lead to fatigue or injury.
- Neglecting to warm up or cool down, increasing the risk of muscle strain.
- Wearing inappropriate footwear, which can cause discomfort or foot problems.

Progress tracking

- Use a pedometer or smartphone app to track your steps and distance.
- Keep a walking journal to note your duration, distance, and how you feel after each session.
- Set weekly goals to gradually increase your walking time and distance.

EXERCISE 3. CHAIR YOGA BASICS

Objective

Introduce chair yoga to enhance flexibility, reduce stress, and support musculoskeletal health.

Step-by-step instructions

- Find a sturdy chair without wheels. Sit with your feet flat on the floor, knees at a 90-degree angle, and back straight.

- Begin with deep breathing. Inhale deeply through your nose, hold for a moment, and exhale slowly through your mouth. Repeat for 3-5 breaths to center your mind.

- Neck stretch: Gently tilt your head to the right, bringing your right ear towards your shoulder. Hold for 5 seconds, then switch to the left side. Repeat 3 times on each side.

- Seated cat-cow: Place your hands on your knees. Inhale, arch your back, and look up (cow pose). Exhale, round your spine, and tuck your chin to your chest (cat pose). Repeat 5 times.

- Seated forward bend: Inhale, lengthen your spine, and as you exhale, hinge at your hips to fold forward, reaching your hands towards the floor. Hold for 5 seconds, then slowly return to the starting position. Repeat 3 times.

- Seated twist: Place your right hand on the back of the chair and your left hand on your right knee. Inhale, lengthen your spine, and as you exhale, gently twist to the right. Hold for 5 seconds, then switch sides. Repeat 3 times on each side.

- Seated leg lift: Extend your right leg straight out, keeping your foot flexed. Hold for 5 seconds, then lower. Repeat 5 times, then switch to the left leg.

- Finish with a relaxation pose: Sit back in your chair, close your eyes, and take slow, deep breaths for 1-2 minutes to relax your body and mind.

Common pitfalls

- Holding your breath during poses, which can increase tension
- Overstretching, which may lead to discomfort or injury
- Using a chair that is unstable or too high, affecting balance

Progress tracking

- Note any improvements in flexibility or reduction in stress levels
- Keep a journal of your practice frequency and any changes in musculoskeletal discomfort
- Set goals to gradually increase the duration or complexity of poses

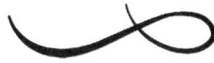

Chapter 8: Three Stress Management Techniques

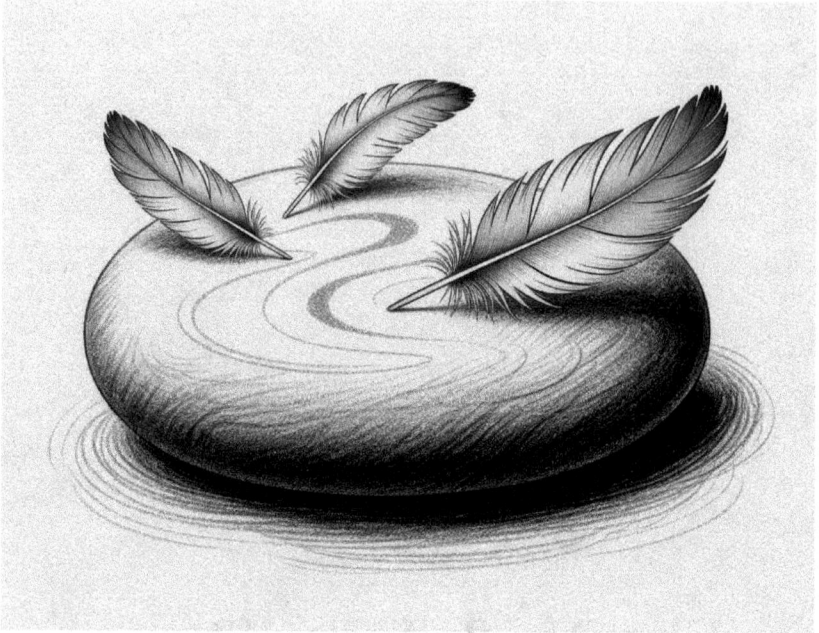

EXERCISE 4. DEEP BREATHING

Objective

Introduce deep breathing techniques to reduce stress, enhance relaxation, and support overall well-being.

Step-by-step instructions

- Find a quiet, comfortable place to sit or lie down. Ensure your back is straight and your body is relaxed.

- Close your eyes gently and place one hand on your chest and the other on your abdomen.

- Inhale slowly through your nose, allowing your abdomen to rise as you fill your lungs with air. Count to four as you inhale.

- Hold your breath for a moment, counting to two.

- Exhale slowly through your mouth, counting to six, and feel your abdomen fall as you release the air.

- Focus on the rhythm of your breath, maintaining a steady, slow pace. Repeat this cycle for 5-10 minutes.

- If your mind wanders, gently bring your focus back to your breath and the sensation of your hands rising and falling.

- Gradually increase the duration of your practice as you become more comfortable with the technique.

Common pitfalls

- Breathing too quickly, which can lead to hyperventilation or dizziness
- Allowing your chest to rise instead of your abdomen, reducing the effectiveness of deep breathing
- Becoming frustrated if your mind wanders, which can increase stress

Progress tracking

- Note any changes in stress levels or relaxation after each session
- Keep a journal of your practice frequency and any improvements in mood or focus
- Set goals to gradually increase the duration of your deep breathing sessions

EXERCISE 5. PROGRESSIVE MUSCLE RELAXATION

Objective

Promote relaxation and reduce stress through the systematic tensing and relaxing of muscle groups.

Step-by-step instructions

- Find a quiet, comfortable place to sit or lie down. Ensure your body is supported and relaxed.

- Close your eyes gently and take a few deep breaths to center your mind.

- Start with your feet. Inhale and tense the muscles in your feet by curling your toes and holding for 5 seconds. Exhale and release the tension, noticing the difference in sensation.

- Move to your calves. Inhale and tighten the muscles in your calves by pointing your toes upward. Hold for 5 seconds, then exhale and relax.

- Continue to your thighs. Inhale and squeeze the muscles in your thighs, holding for 5 seconds. Exhale and let go of the tension.

- Focus on your abdomen. Inhale and contract your abdominal muscles, holding for 5 seconds. Exhale and release.

- Shift to your hands. Inhale and clench your fists tightly for 5 seconds. Exhale and open your hands, feeling the relaxation.

- Move to your arms. Inhale and tense your biceps by bending your elbows and bringing your hands towards your shoulders. Hold for 5 seconds, then exhale and relax.

- Focus on your shoulders. Inhale and lift your shoulders towards your ears, holding for 5 seconds. Exhale and let them drop.

- Finally, focus on your face. Inhale and scrunch your facial muscles, holding for 5 seconds. Exhale and release, allowing your face to soften.

- Take a few deep breaths, noticing the overall relaxation in your body.

Common pitfalls

- Tensing muscles too hard, which can cause discomfort
- Rushing through the exercise, reducing its effectiveness
- Forgetting to breathe deeply, which can increase tension

Progress tracking

- Note any changes in stress levels or relaxation after each session
- Keep a journal of your practice frequency and any improvements in mood or focus
- Set goals to gradually increase the duration of your relaxation sessions

Managing Chronic Diseases: A Practical Guide To Daily Control Of Diabetes, Hypertension, And Musculoskeletal Issues

EXERCISE 6. GUIDED IMAGERY

Objective

Utilize guided imagery to foster a positive mindset, reduce stress, and enhance self-management of chronic conditions

Step-by-step instructions

- Find a quiet, comfortable place to sit or lie down. Ensure your body is relaxed and supported.

- Close your eyes gently and take a few deep breaths to center your mind.

- Imagine a peaceful, safe place where you feel completely at ease. This could be a beach, a forest, or any place that brings you comfort.

- Visualize the details of this place. Notice the colors, sounds, and scents. Engage all your senses to make the image as vivid as possible.

- Picture yourself in this environment, feeling calm and relaxed. Allow any tension or stress to melt away as you immerse yourself in the scene.

- Spend 5-10 minutes in this visualization, focusing on the sensations of peace and tranquility.

- If your mind wanders, gently bring your focus back to the imagery and the feelings of relaxation.

- Gradually bring your awareness back to the present moment. Open your eyes and take a few deep breaths before resuming your day.

Common pitfalls

- Struggling to create a vivid image, which can reduce the effectiveness of the exercise
- Allowing distractions to interrupt the visualization process
- Becoming frustrated if relaxation doesn't occur immediately

Progress tracking

- Note any changes in stress levels or relaxation after each session
- Keep a journal of your practice frequency and any improvements in mood or focus
- Set goals to gradually increase the duration of your guided imagery sessions

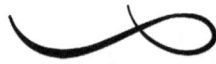

Chapter 9: Tracking Blood Sugar Through Exercise

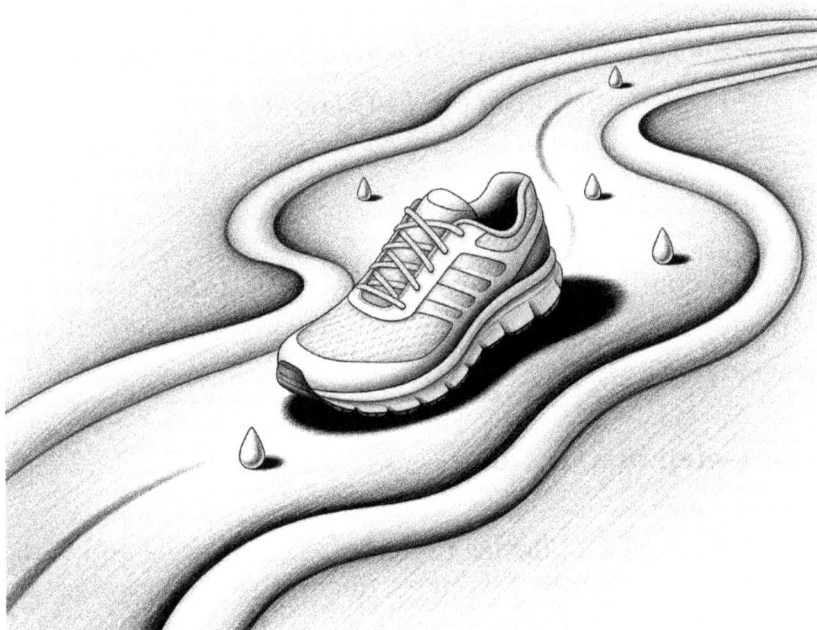

EXERCISE 7. CONTINUOUS GLUCOSE MONITORING SETUP

Objective

Set up a continuous glucose monitoring (CGM) system to effectively track blood sugar levels and enhance diabetes management

Step-by-step instructions

- Choose a CGM device that suits your lifestyle and budget. Consult with your healthcare provider for recommendations.

- Read the user manual thoroughly to understand the device's features and setup process.

- Wash your hands with soap and water to ensure cleanliness before handling the sensor.

- Select a site on your body for sensor placement, typically the abdomen or upper arm. Rotate sites with each new sensor to prevent skin irritation.

- Clean the chosen site with an alcohol wipe and let it dry completely.

- Insert the sensor according to the manufacturer's instructions, using the applicator provided.

- Attach the transmitter to the sensor, ensuring it clicks into place securely.

- Pair the transmitter with your smartphone or receiver device via Bluetooth, following the app's setup instructions.

- Calibrate the CGM if required by your device, using a blood glucose meter for accuracy.

- Set up alerts for high and low blood sugar levels to receive timely notifications.

- Review the data regularly to identify patterns and make informed decisions about your diabetes management.

Common pitfalls

- Failing to rotate sensor sites, leading to skin irritation
- Not calibrating the device as needed, resulting in inaccurate readings
- Ignoring device alerts, which can delay necessary interventions

Progress tracking

- Monitor changes in blood sugar trends over time
- Keep a log of any adjustments made to your diabetes management plan based on CGM data
- Set goals for maintaining target blood sugar ranges and review progress with your healthcare provider

EXERCISE 8. FINGERSTICK TESTING ROUTINE

Objective

Establish a consistent fingerstick testing routine to accurately monitor blood sugar levels and enhance diabetes management

Step-by-step instructions

- Choose a specific time each day for testing, such as before meals or at bedtime, to maintain consistency.

- Wash your hands thoroughly with soap and warm water to ensure cleanliness and accuracy.

- Prepare your testing supplies: glucose meter, test strips, and a lancing device with a new lancet.

- Insert a test strip into the glucose meter, ensuring it is properly aligned.

- Use the lancing device to prick the side of your fingertip, as this area is less sensitive than the pad.

- Gently squeeze your finger to obtain a small drop of blood.

- Touch the edge of the test strip to the blood drop, allowing it to be absorbed.

- Wait for the meter to display your blood sugar reading, which typically takes a few seconds.

- Record the result in a logbook or digital app, noting the time and any relevant details such as food intake or physical activity.

- Dispose of the used lancet and test strip in a sharps container to ensure safe disposal.

Common pitfalls

- Forgetting to wash hands, which can lead to inaccurate readings
- Using expired test strips, resulting in unreliable results
- Not rotating fingers, causing soreness or calluses

Progress tracking

- Keep a detailed log of blood sugar readings to identify patterns and trends
- Review your log with your healthcare provider to adjust your diabetes management plan as needed
- Set goals for maintaining target blood sugar levels and track your progress regularly

EXERCISE 9. BLOOD SUGAR LOG MAINTENANCE

Objective

Maintain an accurate and comprehensive blood sugar log to enhance diabetes management and identify patterns

Step-by-step instructions

- Choose a log format that suits your lifestyle, such as a digital app or a physical notebook.

- Record the date and time of each blood sugar test to track changes throughout the day.

- Note the blood sugar reading immediately after testing to ensure accuracy.

- Include details about meals, snacks, and beverages consumed around the time of testing.

- Document any physical activity, noting the type and duration, as it can impact blood sugar levels.

- Record any medications taken, including the dosage and time, to monitor their effects.

- Add notes on stress levels, sleep quality, or any illness, as these factors can influence blood sugar.

- Review your log weekly to identify trends and patterns in your blood sugar levels.

- Share your log with your healthcare provider during appointments to adjust your management plan as needed.

Common pitfalls

- Forgetting to log immediately after testing, leading to incomplete records
- Omitting details about food intake or physical activity, which can obscure patterns
- Inconsistently recording data, making it difficult to track trends

Progress tracking

- Regularly review your log to assess the effectiveness of your diabetes management plan
- Set specific goals for blood sugar control and monitor your progress over time
- Use your log to facilitate discussions with your healthcare provider about potential adjustments to your treatment plan

EXERCISE 10. ANALYZING BLOOD SUGAR TRENDS

Objective

Identify patterns in blood sugar levels to enhance diabetes management and make informed lifestyle adjustments

Step-by-step instructions

- Gather at least two weeks of blood sugar readings from your logbook or digital app.

- Organize the data by time of day, such as morning, afternoon, and evening readings.

- Calculate the average blood sugar level for each time period to identify typical trends.

- Compare these averages to your target blood sugar range, noting any significant deviations.

- Identify any recurring patterns, such as higher readings after specific meals or activities.

- Consider factors that may influence these patterns, such as diet, exercise, stress, or medication timing.

- Develop a plan to address any identified issues, such as adjusting meal composition or timing of physical activity.

- Implement changes gradually, monitoring their impact on your blood sugar levels over the following weeks.

- Review your findings and adjustments with your healthcare provider to refine your management plan.

Common pitfalls

- Failing to consider all influencing factors, leading to incomplete analysis
- Making too many changes at once, which can obscure the effects of individual adjustments
- Ignoring small deviations that may indicate emerging trends

Progress tracking

- Regularly update your log with new data to continue identifying trends
- Set specific goals for blood sugar control based on identified patterns
- Use your analysis to facilitate discussions with your healthcare provider about potential treatment adjustments

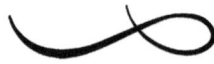

Chapter 10: Monitoring Blood Pressure at Home

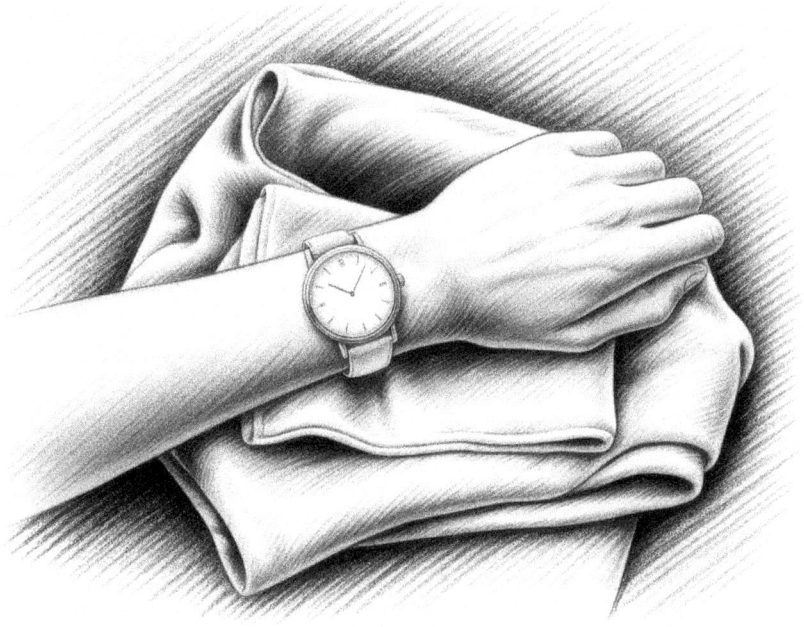

EXERCISE 11. HOME BLOOD PRESSURE CUFF SETUP

Objective

Ensure accurate and consistent blood pressure readings at home to effectively monitor hypertension

Step-by-step instructions

- Choose a reliable blood pressure monitor, preferably an automatic, upper-arm model for accuracy.

- Read the manufacturer's instructions carefully to understand the device's operation and maintenance.

- Select a quiet, comfortable location for measurements, ideally at a table with a chair that supports your back.

- Sit with your feet flat on the floor and your arm supported at heart level on a table.

- Rest for at least 5 minutes before taking a measurement to ensure a calm state.

- Wrap the cuff snugly around your bare upper arm, about 1 inch above the elbow.

- Ensure the cuff's tubing is aligned with the center of your arm and the palm is facing upward.

- Press the start button and remain still and silent while the device measures your blood pressure.

- Record the reading, including the date and time, in a logbook or digital app for tracking.

- Repeat the measurement after 1-2 minutes and average the two readings for accuracy.

Common pitfalls

- Using a cuff that is too small or too large, leading to inaccurate readings
- Taking measurements immediately after eating, exercising, or experiencing stress
- Failing to support the arm at heart level, which can skew results

Progress tracking

- Regularly review your blood pressure log to identify trends and patterns
- Set specific goals for blood pressure control and monitor your progress over time
- Share your log with your healthcare provider to adjust your management plan as needed

EXERCISE 12. PROPER CUFF PLACEMENT

Objective

Ensure the blood pressure cuff is correctly positioned for accurate readings

Step-by-step instructions

- Select a cuff size that fits your arm circumference, typically indicated on the cuff packaging.

- Sit comfortably with your back supported and feet flat on the floor.

- Rest your arm on a table at heart level, palm facing upward.

- Remove any clothing that covers the upper arm to ensure direct contact with the skin.

- Position the cuff on your bare upper arm, about 1 inch above the elbow.

- Align the cuff's tubing with the center of your arm, following the manufacturer's guidelines.

- Wrap the cuff snugly around your arm, ensuring it is neither too tight nor too loose.

- Double-check that the cuff is level with your heart and the tubing is not twisted.

- Proceed with the blood pressure measurement as per the device instructions.

Common pitfalls

- Using a cuff that is not the correct size for your arm, leading to inaccurate readings
- Placing the cuff over clothing, which can interfere with the measurement
- Positioning the cuff too high or too low on the arm, affecting accuracy

Progress tracking

- Regularly review your blood pressure readings to ensure consistency
- Adjust cuff placement if readings are inconsistent or unexpected
- Share your log with your healthcare provider to discuss any necessary adjustments

EXERCISE 13. RECORDING BLOOD PRESSURE READINGS

Objective

Accurately record blood pressure readings to track hypertension management progress

Step-by-step instructions

- Use a consistent method for recording, such as a dedicated notebook or a digital app designed for health tracking.

- Note the date and time of each reading to identify patterns over time.

- Record both systolic and diastolic numbers, as well as the pulse rate if available.

- Include any relevant notes, such as recent activities, stress levels, or dietary factors that might influence the reading.

- Regularly review your log to spot trends, such as consistently high readings at certain times of day.

- Share your records with your healthcare provider during appointments to facilitate informed discussions about your treatment plan.

Common pitfalls

- Forgetting to record readings immediately, leading to inaccurate or incomplete logs
- Failing to note contextual factors that could affect blood pressure, such as stress or caffeine intake
- Inconsistently recording readings, which can obscure trends and hinder effective management

Progress tracking

- Set reminders to take and record readings at the same time each day for consistency
- Use your log to set realistic blood pressure goals and track your progress toward achieving them
- Discuss your records with your healthcare provider to adjust your management plan as needed

EXERCISE 14. ANALYZING BLOOD PRESSURE TRENDS

Objective

Identify patterns in blood pressure readings to enhance self-management and treatment effectiveness

Step-by-step instructions

- Gather at least two weeks of blood pressure readings, ensuring they are taken at consistent times each day.

- Use a graph or chart to plot your systolic and diastolic readings over time, noting the date and time for each entry.

- Look for trends, such as consistently higher readings in the morning or evening, and note any patterns.

- Identify any external factors that may correlate with changes in your readings, such as stress, diet, or physical activity.

- Compare your findings with recommended blood pressure ranges to assess how well your readings align with target levels.

- Use your analysis to adjust lifestyle habits, such as diet or exercise, to better manage your blood pressure.

- Share your findings with your healthcare provider to discuss potential adjustments to your treatment plan.

Common pitfalls

- Failing to record readings consistently, which can obscure trends and hinder analysis
- Overlooking external factors that may influence blood pressure, such as medication changes or stress levels
- Misinterpreting short-term fluctuations as long-term trends

Progress tracking

- Regularly update your chart with new readings to maintain an accurate picture of your blood pressure trends
- Set specific goals based on your analysis, such as reducing stress or increasing physical activity, and track your progress toward achieving them
- Review your trends with your healthcare provider to ensure your management plan remains effective and up-to-date

EXERCISE 15. CREATING A BLOOD PRESSURE LOG

Objective

Develop a personalized blood pressure log to enhance self-monitoring and management

Step-by-step instructions

- Choose a format for your log, such as a paper journal, spreadsheet, or health app, that you find easy to use and access regularly.

- Set a consistent schedule for taking your blood pressure, ideally at the same times each day, such as morning and evening.

- Record each reading immediately, noting the date, time, systolic and diastolic numbers, and pulse rate if available.

- Include additional notes on factors that might affect your readings, such as recent physical activity, stress levels, or dietary choices.

- Review your log weekly to identify any patterns or trends, such as fluctuations related to specific activities or times of day.

- Use your findings to make informed adjustments to your lifestyle, such as modifying your diet or exercise routine, to better manage your blood pressure.

- Share your log with your healthcare provider during appointments to facilitate discussions about your treatment plan and any necessary adjustments.

Common pitfalls

- Inconsistently recording readings, which can lead to an incomplete picture of your blood pressure trends
- Neglecting to note contextual factors that may influence readings, such as stress or caffeine consumption
- Failing to review and analyze your log regularly, missing opportunities for proactive management

Progress tracking

- Set reminders to take and record readings consistently to maintain an accurate log
- Establish specific goals based on your log analysis, such as reducing sodium intake or increasing physical activity, and track your progress
- Regularly discuss your log with your healthcare provider to ensure your management plan remains effective and up-to-date

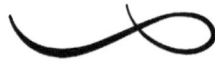

Chapter 11: Setting Realistic Health Goals for Exercise

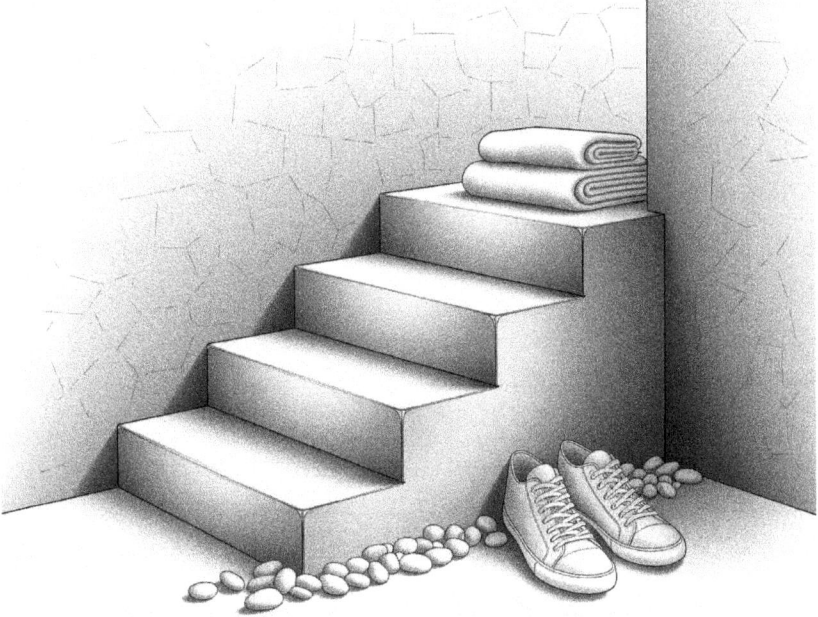

EXERCISE 16. SETTING SMART GOALS

Objective

Create specific, measurable, achievable, relevant, and time-bound goals to enhance chronic disease management

Step-by-step instructions

- Identify a specific area of your health you want to improve, such as lowering blood sugar levels, reducing blood pressure, or increasing physical activity.

- Make your goal measurable by defining clear criteria for success, such as reducing your A1C level by 1% or walking 30 minutes daily.

- Ensure your goal is achievable by considering your current lifestyle and resources. For example, if you're new to exercise, start with a 10-minute walk and gradually increase.

- Confirm that your goal is relevant to your overall health objectives and aligns with your chronic disease management plan.

- Set a time-bound deadline to achieve your goal, such as within three months, to maintain focus and motivation.

- Write down your SMART goal and place it somewhere visible to remind you of your commitment.

- Regularly review your progress and adjust your goal as needed to ensure it remains realistic and aligned with your health needs.

Common pitfalls

- Setting goals that are too vague or broad, making it difficult to measure progress
- Overestimating what can be achieved in a short time, leading to frustration
- Failing to adjust goals when circumstances change, which can hinder progress

Progress tracking

- Use a journal or app to record daily actions and progress toward your goal
- Schedule regular check-ins, such as weekly or bi-weekly, to assess your progress and make necessary adjustments
- Share your goals and progress with a healthcare provider or support group for accountability and encouragement

EXERCISE 17. PRIORITIZING HEALTH OBJECTIVES

Objective

Identify and prioritize health objectives to effectively manage chronic diseases

Step-by-step instructions

- List all health-related goals you wish to achieve, such as improving blood sugar control, reducing joint pain, or lowering blood pressure.

- Rank these goals based on their impact on your overall health and quality of life, considering factors like urgency, feasibility, and personal importance.

- Select the top three goals that align with your current health needs and resources, ensuring they are realistic and achievable.

- Break down each selected goal into smaller, actionable steps that can be integrated into your daily routine.

- Allocate specific timeframes for each step, such as daily, weekly, or monthly, to maintain focus and momentum.

- Regularly review and adjust your priorities as your health status and circumstances evolve, ensuring continued relevance and effectiveness.

Common pitfalls

- Attempting to tackle too many goals at once, leading to overwhelm and reduced effectiveness
- Failing to reassess priorities regularly, which can result in outdated or irrelevant objectives
- Neglecting to consider personal values and lifestyle when setting priorities, reducing motivation

Progress tracking

- Use a planner or digital tool to track progress on each goal and its associated steps
- Schedule regular check-ins, such as monthly, to evaluate progress and make necessary adjustments
- Share your prioritized goals with a healthcare provider or support network for accountability and guidance

EXERCISE 18. TRACKING PROGRESS

Objective

Monitor and evaluate your progress in managing chronic diseases to enhance self-management and motivation

Step-by-step instructions

- Choose a method for tracking your progress, such as a journal, spreadsheet, or mobile app, that fits your lifestyle and preferences.

- Identify key metrics to track based on your health goals, such as blood sugar levels, blood pressure readings, or daily physical activity.

- Set a regular schedule for recording your data, such as daily for blood sugar or weekly for physical activity, to ensure consistency.

- Review your recorded data at the end of each week to identify patterns, improvements, or areas needing attention.

- Adjust your management strategies based on your findings, such as modifying your diet, exercise routine, or medication adherence.

- Share your progress with a healthcare provider or support group to receive feedback and encouragement.

Common pitfalls

- Inconsistent tracking, which can lead to inaccurate assessments of progress
- Focusing solely on negative outcomes, which can decrease motivation
- Neglecting to celebrate small victories, which can reduce overall morale

Progress tracking

- Use visual aids, like graphs or charts, to better understand trends and changes over time
- Set reminders or alarms to prompt regular data entry and review
- Engage with a community or support network to share experiences and gain insights

EXERCISE 19. ADJUSTING GOALS AS NEEDED

Objective

Adapt and refine health goals to ensure they remain achievable
and relevant

Step-by-step instructions

- Review your current health goals and assess their
  progress, considering any changes in your health status
  or lifestyle.

- Identify any obstacles or challenges that have hindered
  your progress, such as time constraints, financial
  limitations, or unexpected health issues.

- Re-evaluate the feasibility of each goal, taking into
  account your current resources, support systems, and
  personal commitments.

- Modify your goals as needed to better align with your
  current situation, ensuring they remain specific,
  measurable, achievable, relevant, and time-bound
  (SMART).

- Break down revised goals into smaller, manageable steps
  that can be easily integrated into your daily routine.

- Set new timeframes for each step, allowing for flexibility
  and adjustments as circumstances change.

- Communicate any changes in your goals with your healthcare provider or support network to receive feedback and encouragement.

Common pitfalls

- Sticking rigidly to original goals despite changing circumstances, leading to frustration and decreased motivation
- Overlooking the need for flexibility and adaptability in goal-setting
- Failing to involve healthcare providers or support networks in the goal adjustment process

Progress tracking

- Use a journal or digital tool to document changes in your goals and track progress on revised steps
- Schedule regular check-ins, such as bi-weekly, to evaluate the effectiveness of adjusted goals
- Share updates with a support group or healthcare provider to maintain accountability and receive guidance

EXERCISE 20. CELEBRATING MILESTONES

Objective

Recognize and celebrate personal achievements in managing chronic diseases to boost motivation and maintain a positive mindset

Step-by-step instructions

- Identify specific milestones related to your health management, such as maintaining stable blood sugar levels for a month, consistently meeting exercise goals, or successfully reducing medication dosage under medical guidance.

- Choose a meaningful way to celebrate each milestone, such as treating yourself to a favorite activity, enjoying a special meal, or taking a day off to relax and recharge.

- Share your achievements with a supportive friend, family member, or support group to enhance the sense of accomplishment and receive encouragement.

- Reflect on the strategies and efforts that led to your success, noting any particular actions or habits that were especially effective.

- Document your milestones and celebrations in a journal or digital tool to create a record of your progress and achievements over time.

- Set new milestones to continue challenging yourself and maintaining momentum in your health management journey.

Common pitfalls

- Overlooking small achievements, which can lead to decreased motivation and morale
- Comparing your progress to others, which can create unnecessary pressure and diminish personal accomplishments
- Failing to acknowledge the effort and dedication required to reach each milestone

Progress tracking

- Use a visual tracker, like a calendar or chart, to mark each milestone and celebration
- Schedule regular reflection sessions to review past achievements and set future goals
- Engage with a support network to share milestones and gain additional motivation

EXERCISE 21. REFLECTING ON ACHIEVEMENTS

Objective

Enhance self-awareness and motivation by reflecting on
personal achievements in managing chronic diseases

Step-by-step instructions

- Set aside a quiet time each week to reflect on your health
  management journey, focusing on both small and
  significant achievements.

- Write down specific instances where you successfully
  managed your condition, such as sticking to a meal plan,
  completing a workout routine, or attending all medical
  appointments.

- Consider the emotions and thoughts you experienced
  during these achievements, noting any positive feelings
  or insights gained.

- Identify the skills, strategies, or support systems that
  contributed to your success, such as time management,
  stress reduction techniques, or encouragement from
  loved ones.

- Acknowledge any challenges you overcame and the
  resilience you demonstrated in facing them.

- Use this reflection to set new, realistic goals that build on
  your achievements and continue to improve your health
  management.

- Share your reflections with a trusted friend, family member, or support group to gain additional perspectives and encouragement.

Common pitfalls

- Focusing only on setbacks or failures, which can overshadow progress and reduce motivation
- Neglecting to recognize the importance of small achievements in the overall journey
- Comparing your journey to others, leading to feelings of inadequacy or discouragement

Progress tracking

- Maintain a dedicated journal or digital document to record reflections and insights regularly
- Review past entries periodically to observe growth and patterns in your health management
- Use visual aids, like charts or graphs, to track progress and highlight achievements over time

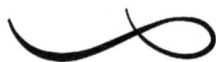

Chapter 12: Creating a Symptom Diary

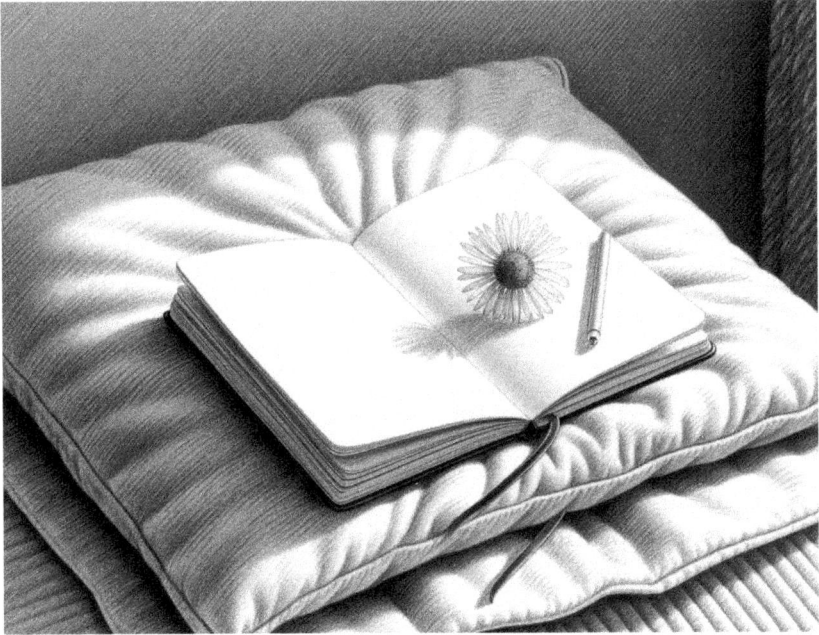

EXERCISE 22. IDENTIFYING SYMPTOMS

Objective

Enhance self-awareness and proactive management by accurately identifying and documenting symptoms related to chronic diseases

Step-by-step instructions

- Choose a dedicated notebook or digital app to serve as your symptom diary, ensuring it is easily accessible for daily entries.

- Set a specific time each day to record your symptoms, such as after breakfast or before bed, to establish a consistent routine.

- Note the date and time of each entry to track patterns and changes over time.

- Describe each symptom in detail, including its intensity, duration, and any potential triggers or alleviating factors.

- Record any related activities, such as meals, physical activity, or stress levels, that may influence your symptoms.

- Use a simple rating scale (e.g., 1-10) to quantify the severity of each symptom for easier comparison and analysis.

- Review your entries weekly to identify trends, improvements, or areas needing attention, and adjust your management strategies accordingly.

- Share your symptom diary with your healthcare provider during appointments to facilitate informed discussions and personalized care plans.

Common pitfalls

- Inconsistent recording, which can lead to incomplete data and hinder pattern recognition
- Overlooking minor symptoms that may provide valuable insights into your condition
- Failing to consider external factors, such as diet or stress, that may impact symptoms

Progress tracking

- Regularly update your symptom diary and review past entries to monitor changes and improvements
- Use visual aids, like graphs or charts, to illustrate symptom patterns and trends over time
- Engage with a support network to discuss findings and gain additional perspectives on symptom management

EXERCISE 23. TRACKING SYMPTOM FREQUENCY

Objective

Enhance understanding of symptom patterns by consistently tracking the frequency of symptoms related to chronic diseases

Step-by-step instructions

- Select a dedicated notebook or digital tool to log symptom frequency, ensuring it is easily accessible for daily use.

- Establish a routine by choosing a specific time each day to record symptoms, such as after breakfast or before bed.

- Note the date and time of each entry to maintain a chronological record.

- List each symptom you experience, noting how often it occurs throughout the day.

- Use a simple tally system or checkmarks to count occurrences, making it easy to visualize frequency.

- Record any activities, meals, or stressors that coincide with symptom occurrences to identify potential triggers.

- Review your entries weekly to detect patterns or changes in symptom frequency, adjusting management strategies as needed.

- Share your findings with your healthcare provider to support informed discussions and personalized care plans.

Common pitfalls

- Inconsistent logging, which can obscure patterns and hinder effective management
- Ignoring minor symptoms that may provide valuable insights into your condition
- Failing to consider external factors, such as diet or stress, that may influence symptom frequency

Progress tracking

- Regularly update your symptom log and review past entries to monitor changes and improvements
- Use visual aids, like graphs or charts, to illustrate symptom frequency and trends over time
- Engage with a support network to discuss findings and gain additional perspectives on symptom management

EXERCISE 24. NOTING SYMPTOM DURATION

Objective

Improve symptom management by accurately tracking the duration of symptoms related to chronic diseases

Step-by-step instructions

- Choose a dedicated notebook or digital app to serve as your symptom diary, ensuring it is easily accessible for daily entries.

- Set a specific time each day to record your symptoms, such as after breakfast or before bed, to establish a consistent routine.

- Note the date and time of each entry to track patterns and changes over time.

- For each symptom, record the start and end time to determine its duration.

- Describe the symptom in detail, including its intensity and any potential triggers or alleviating factors.

- Record any related activities, such as meals, physical activity, or stress levels, that may influence your symptoms.

- Use a simple rating scale (e.g., 1-10) to quantify the severity of each symptom for easier comparison and analysis.

- Review your entries weekly to identify trends, improvements, or areas needing attention, and adjust your management strategies accordingly.

- Share your symptom diary with your healthcare provider during appointments to facilitate informed discussions and personalized care plans

Common pitfalls

- Inconsistent recording, which can lead to incomplete data and hinder pattern recognition
- Overlooking minor symptoms that may provide valuable insights into your condition
- Failing to consider external factors, such as diet or stress, that may impact symptoms

Progress tracking

- Regularly update your symptom diary and review past entries to monitor changes and improvements
- Use visual aids, like graphs or charts, to illustrate symptom patterns and trends over time
- Engage with a support network to discuss findings and gain additional perspectives on symptom management

EXERCISE 25. RECORDING SYMPTOM INTENSITY

Objective

Enhance understanding of symptom intensity by consistently tracking the severity of symptoms related to chronic diseases

Step-by-step instructions

- Choose a dedicated notebook or digital app to serve as your symptom diary, ensuring it is easily accessible for daily entries.

- Set a specific time each day to record your symptoms, such as after breakfast or before bed, to establish a consistent routine.

- Note the date and time of each entry to track patterns and changes over time.

- For each symptom, use a simple rating scale (e.g., 1-10) to quantify its intensity, with 1 being very mild and 10 being extremely severe.

- Describe the symptom in detail, including any potential triggers or alleviating factors.

- Record any related activities, such as meals, physical activity, or stress levels, that may influence your symptoms.

- Review your entries weekly to identify trends, improvements, or areas needing attention, and adjust your management strategies accordingly.

- Share your symptom diary with your healthcare provider during appointments to facilitate informed discussions and personalized care plans

Common pitfalls

- Inconsistent recording, which can lead to incomplete data and hinder pattern recognition
- Overlooking minor symptoms that may provide valuable insights into your condition
- Failing to consider external factors, such as diet or stress, that may impact symptoms

Progress tracking

- Regularly update your symptom diary and review past entries to monitor changes and improvements
- Use visual aids, like graphs or charts, to illustrate symptom patterns and trends over time
- Engage with a support network to discuss findings and gain additional perspectives on symptom management

EXERCISE 26. DOCUMENTING SYMPTOM TRIGGERS

Objective

Identify and understand the triggers of symptoms related to chronic diseases for better management and prevention

Step-by-step instructions

- Select a dedicated notebook or digital app to serve as your symptom diary, ensuring it is easily accessible for daily entries.

- Establish a consistent time each day to document your symptoms, such as after breakfast or before bed.

- Record the date and time of each entry to track patterns and changes over time.

- For each symptom, describe it in detail, including its intensity and any potential triggers or alleviating factors.

- Note any activities, such as meals, physical activity, or stress levels, that occurred before the onset of symptoms.

- Identify and record any environmental factors, such as weather changes or exposure to allergens, that may influence your symptoms.

- Use a simple rating scale (e.g., 1-10) to quantify the severity of each symptom for easier comparison and analysis.

- Review your entries weekly to identify trends, improvements, or areas needing attention, and adjust your management strategies accordingly.

- Share your symptom diary with your healthcare provider during appointments to facilitate informed discussions and personalized care plans

Common pitfalls

- Inconsistent recording, which can lead to incomplete data and hinder pattern recognition
- Overlooking minor symptoms that may provide valuable insights into your condition
- Failing to consider external factors, such as diet or stress, that may impact symptoms

Progress tracking

- Regularly update your symptom diary and review past entries to monitor changes and improvements
- Use visual aids, like graphs or charts, to illustrate symptom patterns and trends over time
- Engage with a support network to discuss findings and gain additional perspectives on symptom management

EXERCISE 27. LOGGING SYMPTOM RELIEF METHODS

Objective

Identify and document effective methods for alleviating symptoms related to chronic diseases

Step-by-step instructions

- Choose a dedicated notebook or digital app to serve as your symptom relief log, ensuring it is easily accessible for daily entries.

- Set a specific time each day to record your symptom relief methods, such as after breakfast or before bed, to establish a consistent routine.

- Note the date and time of each entry to track patterns and changes over time.

- For each symptom, describe the relief method used, including any medications, exercises, dietary changes, or relaxation techniques.

- Use a simple rating scale (e.g., 1-10) to quantify the effectiveness of each relief method, with 1 being not effective and 10 being highly effective.

- Record any side effects or additional benefits experienced from the relief method.

- Note any related activities, such as meals, physical activity, or stress levels, that may influence the effectiveness of the relief method.

- Review your entries weekly to identify the most effective relief methods and adjust your management strategies accordingly.

- Share your symptom relief log with your healthcare provider during appointments to facilitate informed discussions and personalized care plans

Common pitfalls

- Inconsistent recording, which can lead to incomplete data and hinder pattern recognition
- Overlooking minor relief methods that may provide valuable insights into your condition
- Failing to consider external factors, such as diet or stress, that may impact the effectiveness of relief methods

Progress tracking

- Regularly update your symptom relief log and review past entries to monitor changes and improvements
- Use visual aids, like graphs or charts, to illustrate the effectiveness of relief methods over time
- Engage with a support network to discuss findings and gain additional perspectives on symptom management

EXERCISE 28. REVIEWING SYMPTOM PATTERNS

Objective

Identify and analyze patterns in symptoms to enhance self-management and improve quality of life

Step-by-step instructions

- Gather your symptom diary entries from the past month, ensuring all relevant data is included for comprehensive analysis.

- Create a table or spreadsheet to organize your entries, categorizing them by date, symptom type, intensity, and potential triggers.

- Use color-coding or symbols to highlight recurring symptoms and their associated triggers for easier visualization.

- Identify any patterns or correlations between symptoms and specific activities, foods, or environmental factors.

- Note any time of day or week when symptoms are more prevalent, considering lifestyle factors that may contribute.

- Compare symptom patterns with your daily routines, such as diet, exercise, and stress levels, to identify potential areas for adjustment.

- Develop a list of potential changes to your daily routine based on identified patterns, focusing on reducing symptom frequency and intensity.

- Implement one change at a time, allowing at least two weeks to assess its impact on your symptoms.

- Document any changes in symptom patterns after implementing adjustments, noting improvements or new insights.

- Share your findings and proposed changes with your healthcare provider to refine your management plan and receive professional guidance

Common pitfalls

- Failing to review entries regularly, which can delay pattern recognition and necessary adjustments
- Overlooking subtle patterns that may provide valuable insights into symptom management
- Making multiple changes simultaneously, which can complicate the identification of effective strategies

Progress tracking

- Regularly update your symptom diary and review entries to monitor changes and improvements
- Use visual aids, like graphs or charts, to illustrate symptom patterns and the impact of implemented changes
- Engage with a support network to discuss findings and gain additional perspectives on symptom management

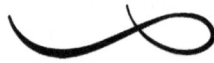

Chapter 13: Improving Sleep Hygiene Through Exercise

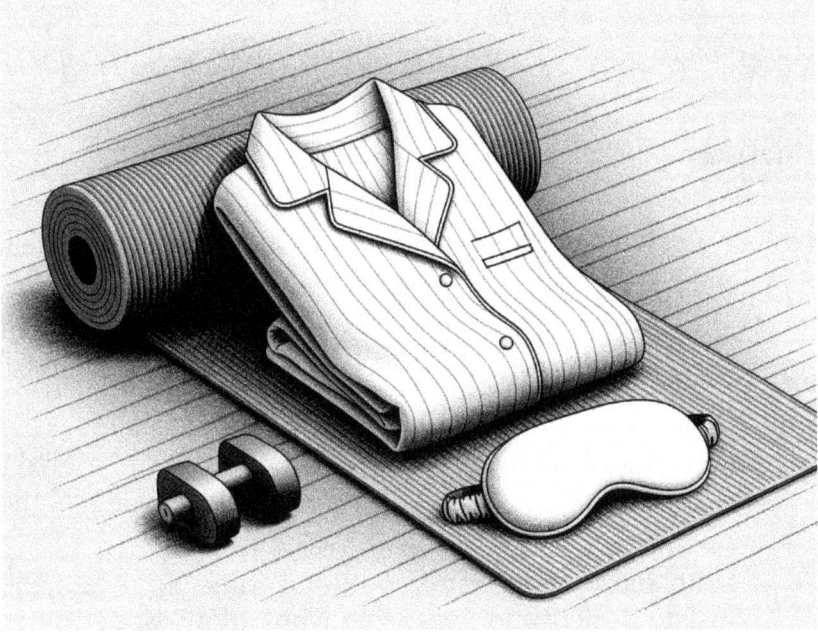

EXERCISE 29. ESTABLISHING A SLEEP SCHEDULE

Objective

Establish a consistent sleep schedule to improve overall health and manage chronic conditions effectively

Step-by-step instructions

- Determine your ideal wake-up time based on your daily commitments and aim for 7-9 hours of sleep each night.

- Count back from your wake-up time to establish a consistent bedtime, ensuring you allow time to wind down before sleep.

- Set an alarm for both your wake-up time and bedtime to reinforce your new schedule.

- Create a relaxing pre-sleep routine, such as reading or taking a warm bath, to signal your body that it's time to wind down.

- Avoid screens, caffeine, and heavy meals at least one hour before bedtime to promote better sleep quality.

- Keep your sleep environment comfortable, cool, and dark, using blackout curtains or a sleep mask if necessary.

- Limit naps to 20-30 minutes and avoid napping late in the day to maintain your sleep schedule.

- Gradually adjust your sleep schedule by 15-30 minutes each day if needed, to reach your desired bedtime and wake-up time.

- Track your sleep patterns and any changes in your symptoms to assess the impact of your new schedule on your chronic condition management.

Common pitfalls

- Inconsistency in sleep and wake times, which can disrupt your body's natural rhythm
- Engaging in stimulating activities before bed, making it harder to fall asleep
- Ignoring environmental factors, such as noise or light, that may affect sleep quality

Progress tracking

- Use a sleep diary or app to monitor your sleep duration and quality
- Note any improvements in energy levels, mood, or symptom management
- Share your sleep data with your healthcare provider to discuss potential adjustments to your management plan

EXERCISE 30. CREATING A RELAXING BEDTIME ROUTINE

Objective

Establish a calming bedtime routine to enhance sleep quality and support chronic disease management

Step-by-step instructions

- Choose a consistent time to begin your bedtime routine, ideally 30-60 minutes before your desired sleep time.

- Dim the lights in your home to signal your body that it's time to wind down.

- Engage in a calming activity, such as reading a book, listening to soothing music, or practicing gentle yoga or meditation.

- Avoid stimulating activities, including watching TV, using electronic devices, or engaging in intense conversations.

- Prepare a warm, caffeine-free beverage, like herbal tea, to help relax your body and mind.

- Take a warm bath or shower to help lower your body temperature, which can promote better sleep.

- Practice deep breathing exercises or progressive muscle relaxation to release tension and stress.

- Ensure your bedroom environment is conducive to sleep by keeping it cool, quiet, and dark.

- Use a white noise machine or earplugs if necessary to block out disruptive sounds.

- Reflect on positive moments from your day or write in a gratitude journal to cultivate a peaceful mindset before sleep

Common pitfalls

- Skipping the routine due to time constraints, which can disrupt sleep quality
- Engaging in activities that are too stimulating, making it difficult to relax
- Neglecting to create a sleep-friendly environment, impacting overall restfulness

Progress tracking

- Keep a journal to note any changes in sleep quality and how you feel upon waking
- Monitor improvements in your chronic condition symptoms as your sleep routine becomes established
- Share your observations with your healthcare provider to discuss any necessary adjustments

EXERCISE 31. LIMITING CAFFEINE AND ALCOHOL INTAKE

Objective

Reduce caffeine and alcohol consumption to support effective self-management of chronic conditions

Step-by-step instructions

- Identify your current caffeine and alcohol intake by keeping a detailed log for one week, noting the type and amount of each beverage consumed.

- Set realistic reduction goals, such as limiting caffeine to no more than 400 mg per day (about four 8-ounce cups of brewed coffee) and alcohol to no more than one drink per day for women and two for men.

- Gradually decrease your caffeine intake by substituting one caffeinated beverage per day with a caffeine-free alternative, like herbal tea or water.

- Choose specific days or occasions to enjoy alcohol, and replace other instances with non-alcoholic options, such as sparkling water with a splash of juice.

- Avoid consuming caffeine and alcohol at least 4-6 hours before bedtime to improve sleep quality and reduce the impact on your chronic condition.

- Experiment with different caffeine-free and non-alcoholic beverages to find enjoyable alternatives that satisfy your taste preferences.

- Monitor your body's response to reduced caffeine and alcohol intake, noting any improvements in symptoms, energy levels, or sleep quality.

- Share your progress and any challenges with a healthcare provider to receive personalized advice and support.

Common pitfalls

- Abruptly cutting out caffeine or alcohol, which can lead to withdrawal symptoms or increased cravings
- Replacing caffeinated or alcoholic beverages with sugary or high-calorie alternatives, which may negatively impact health
- Underestimating the caffeine content in certain foods and medications

Progress tracking

- Maintain a journal to record your daily caffeine and alcohol consumption and any changes in your chronic condition symptoms
- Use a mobile app to track your intake and set reminders for your reduction goals
- Discuss your progress with a healthcare provider to evaluate the impact on your overall health and adjust your management plan as needed

EXERCISE 32. OPTIMIZING SLEEP ENVIRONMENT

Objective

Create an optimal sleep environment to enhance rest and support chronic disease management

Step-by-step instructions

- Set your bedroom temperature between 60-67°F to promote comfortable sleep.

- Invest in a quality mattress and pillows that provide adequate support for your body, especially if you have musculoskeletal issues.

- Use blackout curtains or an eye mask to block out light and maintain darkness.

- Remove electronic devices from the bedroom to minimize distractions and blue light exposure.

- Choose calming colors for your bedroom decor, such as soft blues or greens, to create a soothing atmosphere.

- Incorporate calming scents, like lavender or chamomile, using essential oils or a diffuser.

- Keep your bedroom organized and clutter-free to reduce stress and promote relaxation.

- Ensure your bedding is clean and comfortable, using breathable fabrics like cotton or bamboo.

- Limit noise by using a white noise machine or earplugs to block out disruptive sounds.

- Regularly ventilate your bedroom to maintain fresh air and reduce allergens.

Common pitfalls

- Overlooking the importance of a supportive mattress and pillows, which can exacerbate musculoskeletal discomfort
- Neglecting to remove electronic devices, leading to disrupted sleep patterns
- Failing to maintain a consistent sleep environment, impacting overall sleep quality

Progress tracking

- Keep a sleep diary to record changes in sleep quality and duration
- Note any improvements in chronic condition symptoms as your sleep environment becomes optimized
- Discuss your observations with a healthcare provider to make any necessary adjustments

EXERCISE 33. PRACTICING MINDFUL BREATHING BEFORE BED

Objective

Enhance relaxation and improve sleep quality through mindful breathing techniques

Step-by-step instructions

- Find a comfortable position in your bed, lying on your back with your arms resting at your sides or on your abdomen.

- Close your eyes gently and take a deep breath in through your nose, allowing your abdomen to rise as you fill your lungs with air.

- Hold your breath for a count of four, feeling the fullness of your breath.

- Slowly exhale through your mouth, letting your abdomen fall as you release the air completely.

- Continue this breathing pattern, inhaling for a count of four, holding for a count of four, and exhaling for a count of four.

- Focus your attention on the sensation of your breath, noticing the rise and fall of your abdomen and the flow of air in and out of your body.

- If your mind begins to wander, gently bring your focus back to your breath without judgment.

- Practice this mindful breathing for 5-10 minutes, gradually increasing the duration as you become more comfortable with the technique.

Common pitfalls

- Allowing distractions to interrupt your focus, which can reduce the effectiveness of the exercise
- Breathing too quickly or shallowly, which may increase tension rather than promote relaxation

Progress tracking

- Keep a journal to note any changes in sleep quality and overall relaxation
- Record any improvements in chronic condition symptoms as a result of regular mindful breathing practice
- Discuss your experiences with a healthcare provider to tailor the technique to your specific needs

EXERCISE 34. JOURNALING TO CLEAR THE MIND

Objective

Develop a positive mindset and enhance self-management through regular journaling

Step-by-step instructions

- Choose a dedicated notebook or digital app for your journaling practice to keep your entries organized and easily accessible.

- Set aside 10-15 minutes each day, preferably at the same time, to establish a consistent journaling routine.

- Begin each entry by noting the date and time to track your progress and identify patterns over time.

- Start with a brief reflection on your current mood and any physical sensations you are experiencing, such as tension or relaxation.

- Write about any challenges or successes you encountered in managing your chronic condition that day, focusing on specific events or interactions.

- Explore your thoughts and feelings about these experiences, considering how they impact your overall well-being and self-management efforts.

- Conclude each entry with a positive affirmation or intention for the next day, reinforcing a supportive mindset.

- Review past entries weekly to identify recurring themes or insights that can inform your self-management strategies.

Common pitfalls

- Skipping journaling sessions due to time constraints, which can disrupt the habit and reduce its effectiveness
- Focusing solely on negative experiences, which may hinder the development of a positive mindset

Progress tracking

- Note any changes in your emotional well-being and self-management effectiveness over time
- Record improvements in chronic condition symptoms as a result of regular journaling practice
- Share your insights with a healthcare provider to enhance your self-management plan

EXERCISE 35. USING WHITE NOISE FOR BETTER SLEEP

Objective

Enhance sleep quality and relaxation through the use of white noise

Step-by-step instructions

- Choose a white noise source, such as a white noise machine, smartphone app, or online streaming service.

- Set the volume to a comfortable level, ensuring it is loud enough to mask disruptive sounds but not so loud that it becomes a distraction.

- Position the white noise source at a distance from your bed that allows for even sound distribution throughout the room.

- Select a white noise setting that you find soothing, such as rain, ocean waves, or a steady fan sound.

- Turn on the white noise 15-30 minutes before bedtime to help signal to your body that it is time to wind down.

- Allow the white noise to play continuously throughout the night to maintain a consistent auditory environment.

- Experiment with different white noise settings and volumes to find the combination that best supports your sleep.

- If using a smartphone app, ensure your device is set to "Do Not Disturb" mode to prevent interruptions from notifications.

Common pitfalls

- Choosing a white noise setting that is too stimulating, which can hinder relaxation
- Setting the volume too high, which may cause discomfort or disrupt sleep

Progress tracking

- Keep a sleep journal to note any changes in sleep quality and duration
- Record any improvements in chronic condition symptoms as a result of using white noise
- Discuss your experiences with a healthcare provider to tailor the use of white noise to your specific needs

EXERCISE 36. PROGRESSIVE RELAXATION FOR SLEEP

Objective

Enhance relaxation and improve sleep quality through progressive muscle relaxation

Step-by-step instructions

- Find a quiet, comfortable space where you can lie down or sit without distractions.

- Close your eyes and take a few deep breaths, inhaling through your nose and exhaling through your mouth.

- Begin with your toes, tensing the muscles for 5 seconds, then slowly releasing the tension for 10 seconds.

- Move to your calves, tensing the muscles for 5 seconds, then releasing for 10 seconds.

- Continue this pattern, working your way up through your thighs, abdomen, chest, arms, and shoulders.

- Focus on each muscle group, tensing for 5 seconds and releasing for 10 seconds, while maintaining deep, steady breathing.

- Once you reach your shoulders, tense your neck and face muscles, then release.

- After completing the sequence, take a few moments to notice the relaxation throughout your body.

Common pitfalls

- Rushing through the exercise, which can reduce its effectiveness
- Holding your breath while tensing muscles, which may cause discomfort

Progress tracking

- Keep a sleep journal to note any changes in sleep quality and duration
- Record any improvements in chronic condition symptoms as a result of regular practice
- Share your experiences with a healthcare provider to tailor the exercise to your specific needs

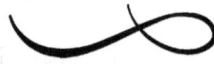

Chapter 14: Building a Daily Exercise Routine

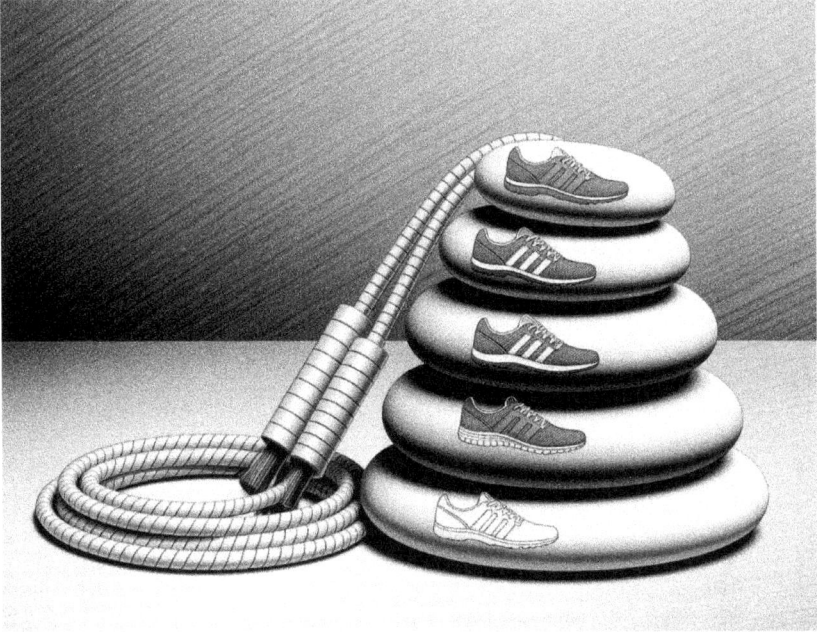

EXERCISE 37. MORNING STRETCH ROUTINE

Objective

Promote flexibility and reduce stiffness to support musculoskeletal health

Step-by-step instructions

- Begin by standing with your feet shoulder-width apart, arms relaxed at your sides.

- Inhale deeply, raising your arms overhead, and stretch your fingertips toward the ceiling.

- Exhale slowly, bending forward at the hips, and let your arms hang toward the floor. Hold for 10 seconds.

- Return to standing, then gently roll your shoulders backward in a circular motion 5 times.

- Extend your right arm across your chest, using your left hand to gently press it closer to your body. Hold for 15 seconds, then switch arms.

- Stand on your left leg, bending your right knee to bring your heel toward your glutes. Hold your right ankle with your right hand for 15 seconds, then switch legs.

- Place your hands on your hips and gently twist your torso to the right, holding for 10 seconds. Repeat on the left side.

- Finish by standing tall, taking a deep breath, and slowly exhaling while relaxing your shoulders.

Common pitfalls

- Skipping the warm-up, which can increase the risk of injury
- Overstretching, which may cause discomfort or strain

Progress tracking

- Keep a journal to note any improvements in flexibility and reduction in stiffness
- Record any changes in chronic condition symptoms as a result of regular stretching
- Share your progress with a healthcare provider to adjust the routine as needed

EXERCISE 38. HYDRATION TRACKING

Objective

Improve hydration levels to support overall health and manage chronic conditions

Step-by-step instructions

- Begin your day by drinking a glass of water (8 oz) upon waking to kickstart hydration.

- Set a daily water intake goal based on your weight: aim for half your body weight in ounces (e.g., if you weigh 160 lbs, target 80 oz of water).

- Use a reusable water bottle with measurement markings to track your intake throughout the day.

- Schedule water breaks: drink a glass of water (8 oz) every 2-3 hours, aligning with meals and snacks.

- Incorporate hydrating foods like cucumbers, watermelon, and oranges into your meals and snacks.

- Monitor the color of your urine: aim for a light, pale yellow as an indicator of proper hydration.

- Set reminders on your phone or use a hydration app to prompt regular water consumption.

- Adjust your water intake based on activity level and climate, increasing consumption during exercise or in hot weather.

Common pitfalls

- Relying solely on thirst as an indicator, which may lead to underhydration
- Consuming excessive caffeinated or sugary beverages, which can contribute to dehydration

Progress tracking

- Keep a daily log of your water intake and note any changes in energy levels or symptoms
- Share your hydration progress with a healthcare provider to ensure it aligns with your health needs

EXERCISE 39. BALANCED MEAL PREPARATION

Objective

Create balanced meals to support chronic disease management
and improve overall health

Step-by-step instructions

- Begin by planning your meals for the week, focusing on
  incorporating a variety of food groups: lean proteins,
  whole grains, fruits, vegetables, and healthy fats.

- Use a plate method for portion control: fill half your plate
  with non-starchy vegetables, one-quarter with lean
  protein, and one-quarter with whole grains or starchy
  vegetables.

- Choose lean protein sources such as chicken, fish, tofu, or
  legumes, aiming for 3-4 ounces per meal.

- Select whole grains like brown rice, quinoa, or whole
  wheat pasta, measuring about 1/2 cup per serving.

- Incorporate a variety of colorful vegetables, aiming for at
  least 2-3 different types per meal to ensure a range of
  nutrients.

- Add healthy fats in moderation, such as a tablespoon of
  olive oil, a quarter of an avocado, or a small handful of
  nuts.

- Limit added sugars and sodium by preparing meals at home and using herbs and spices for flavor instead of salt.

- Stay hydrated by drinking water with meals and throughout the day, avoiding sugary drinks.

Common pitfalls

- Skipping meal planning, which can lead to unhealthy food choices
- Overeating due to large portion sizes or lack of portion control

Progress tracking

- Keep a food diary to monitor meal composition and portion sizes
- Note any changes in energy levels, weight, or chronic condition symptoms
- Share your meal plans and progress with a healthcare provider for personalized feedback

EXERCISE 40. MIDDAY WALK

Objective

Incorporate a midday walk to enhance physical activity, reduce stress, and support chronic disease management

Step-by-step instructions

- Schedule a 15-30 minute walk during your lunch break or midday pause, aiming for at least 5 days a week.

- Choose a safe, accessible route near your workplace or home, such as a park, quiet street, or indoor mall.

- Wear comfortable walking shoes and dress appropriately for the weather to ensure a pleasant experience.

- Begin with a 5-minute warm-up, walking at a leisurely pace to prepare your muscles and joints.

- Gradually increase your pace to a brisk walk, maintaining a speed that elevates your heart rate but allows for conversation.

- Focus on maintaining good posture: keep your head up, shoulders relaxed, and arms swinging naturally.

- Use this time to clear your mind, practice deep breathing, or listen to music or a podcast for motivation.

- Cool down with a 5-minute slow walk, followed by gentle stretching to prevent stiffness and improve flexibility.

Common pitfalls

- Skipping the walk due to workload or time constraints
- Walking too fast or too slow, which may reduce the effectiveness of the exercise

Progress tracking

- Keep a log of your walking sessions, noting duration, distance, and any changes in mood or energy levels
- Share your walking routine with a healthcare provider to ensure it aligns with your health goals

EXERCISE 41. AFTERNOON RELAXATION TECHNIQUES

Objective

Incorporate afternoon relaxation techniques to reduce stress, enhance mental clarity, and support chronic disease management

Step-by-step instructions

- Set aside 10-15 minutes in the afternoon for relaxation, ideally between 2:00 PM and 4:00 PM, when energy levels typically dip.

- Find a quiet, comfortable space where you can sit or lie down without distractions.

- Begin with deep breathing exercises: inhale slowly through your nose for a count of four, hold for four, and exhale through your mouth for a count of four. Repeat for 3-5 minutes.

- Practice progressive muscle relaxation by tensing and then relaxing each muscle group, starting from your toes and working up to your head.

- Engage in a brief mindfulness meditation: focus on your breath, gently bringing your attention back whenever your mind wanders.

- Consider using a guided relaxation app or soothing music to enhance the experience.

- Conclude with gentle stretching, focusing on areas prone to tension such as the neck, shoulders, and back.

Common pitfalls

- Skipping relaxation due to a busy schedule or feeling guilty about taking a break
- Allowing distractions like phone notifications or background noise to interrupt the session

Progress tracking

- Keep a relaxation journal to note the frequency of sessions and any changes in stress levels or symptoms
- Share your relaxation routine with a healthcare provider to discuss its impact on your overall health

EXERCISE 42. EVENING STRETCH ROUTINE

Objective

Incorporate an evening stretch routine to enhance flexibility, reduce muscle tension, and support chronic disease management

Step-by-step instructions

- Set aside 10-15 minutes in the evening, ideally after dinner or before bedtime, to perform your stretch routine.

- Find a quiet, comfortable space with enough room to move freely, such as a living room or bedroom.

- Begin with a gentle warm-up: march in place or perform light arm circles for 2-3 minutes to increase blood flow.

- Perform a standing quadriceps stretch: stand on one leg, bend the opposite knee, and bring your heel towards your buttocks. Hold for 15-30 seconds, then switch legs.

- Execute a seated hamstring stretch: sit on the floor with one leg extended and the other bent. Reach towards your toes, keeping your back straight. Hold for 15-30 seconds, then switch legs.

- Engage in a cat-cow stretch: position yourself on all fours, arch your back upwards (cat), then lower it while lifting your head and tailbone (cow). Repeat 5-10 times.

- Perform a seated spinal twist: sit with legs extended, bend one knee, and place the foot outside the opposite thigh. Twist your torso towards the bent knee, holding for 15-30 seconds, then switch sides.

- Conclude with a deep breathing exercise: sit or lie down comfortably, inhale deeply through your nose, hold for a moment, and exhale slowly through your mouth. Repeat for 3-5 minutes.

Common pitfalls

- Skipping the routine due to fatigue or lack of time
- Overstretching, which may lead to discomfort or injury

Progress tracking

- Maintain a log of your stretching sessions, noting any improvements in flexibility or reduction in muscle tension
- Discuss your stretching routine with a healthcare provider to ensure it complements your overall health plan

EXERCISE 43. DAILY MEDICATION CHECKLIST

Objective

Ensure consistent and accurate medication intake to effectively manage chronic diseases and improve overall health

Step-by-step instructions

- Create a comprehensive list of all medications, including prescription drugs, over-the-counter medications, and supplements. Note the name, dosage, and frequency for each.

- Designate a specific time each day for taking medications, aligning with your daily routine to enhance consistency. Consider using meal times or bedtime as reminders.

- Use a pill organizer with compartments for each day of the week to pre-sort medications, reducing the risk of missed doses or errors.

- Set alarms or reminders on your phone or a digital device to prompt you when it's time to take your medications.

- Keep a medication log to track each dose taken, noting the time and any side effects or symptoms experienced.

- Regularly review your medication list with your healthcare provider to ensure all prescriptions are current and necessary.

- Store medications in a cool, dry place, away from direct sunlight and out of reach of children and pets.

Common pitfalls

- Forgetting to take medications due to a busy schedule or distractions
- Running out of medications without a plan for refills

Progress tracking

- Maintain a medication journal to record adherence and any changes in symptoms or side effects
- Share your medication log with your healthcare provider to discuss its impact on your health management plan

EXERCISE 44. SYMPTOM JOURNAL UPDATE

Objective

Maintain an up-to-date symptom journal to enhance self-awareness and improve communication with healthcare providers

Step-by-step instructions

- Choose a format for your symptom journal, such as a notebook, digital app, or spreadsheet, that fits your lifestyle and preferences.

- Set aside a specific time each day, such as after dinner or before bed, to update your journal consistently.

- Record the date and time of each entry to track patterns and changes over time.

- Note any symptoms experienced, including their intensity, duration, and any potential triggers or alleviating factors.

- Include details about your daily activities, diet, medication intake, and stress levels to identify correlations with symptom changes.

- Review your journal entries weekly to identify trends or recurring issues that may require attention or adjustment in your management plan.

- Share your symptom journal with your healthcare provider during appointments to facilitate informed discussions and personalized care adjustments.

Common pitfalls

- Inconsistent journaling, leading to incomplete data and missed patterns
- Overlooking minor symptoms that may provide valuable insights

Progress tracking

- Regularly assess your symptom journal for improvements or worsening of symptoms
- Use insights from your journal to make informed decisions about lifestyle adjustments and treatment options

EXERCISE 45. EVENING REFLECTION AND PLANNING

Objective

Cultivate a positive mindset and enhance self-management skills by reflecting on daily experiences and planning for the next day

Step-by-step instructions

- Set aside 10-15 minutes each evening in a quiet space to focus on reflection and planning.

- Begin by taking a few deep breaths to center yourself and clear your mind of distractions.

- Reflect on the day's events, considering both positive experiences and challenges faced. Note any specific moments that impacted your mood or health management.

- Identify one or two positive outcomes or achievements from the day, no matter how small, and acknowledge your efforts in achieving them.

- Consider any challenges or setbacks encountered, and think about what you learned from these experiences. Identify any patterns or triggers that may have influenced these situations.

- Plan for the next day by setting one or two realistic goals related to managing your chronic condition, such as trying a new healthy recipe or scheduling time for physical activity.

- Write down your reflections and plans in a journal or digital app to track your progress and maintain accountability.

- Conclude the session by visualizing a successful and positive day ahead, reinforcing your commitment to self-care and effective management.

Common pitfalls

- Skipping reflection time due to fatigue or a busy schedule
- Focusing solely on negative experiences without acknowledging positive aspects

Progress tracking

- Review your journal entries weekly to assess progress and identify areas for improvement
- Share insights with a trusted friend or healthcare provider to gain additional support and perspective

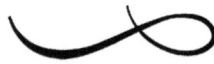

Chapter 15: Communicating with Healthcare Providers

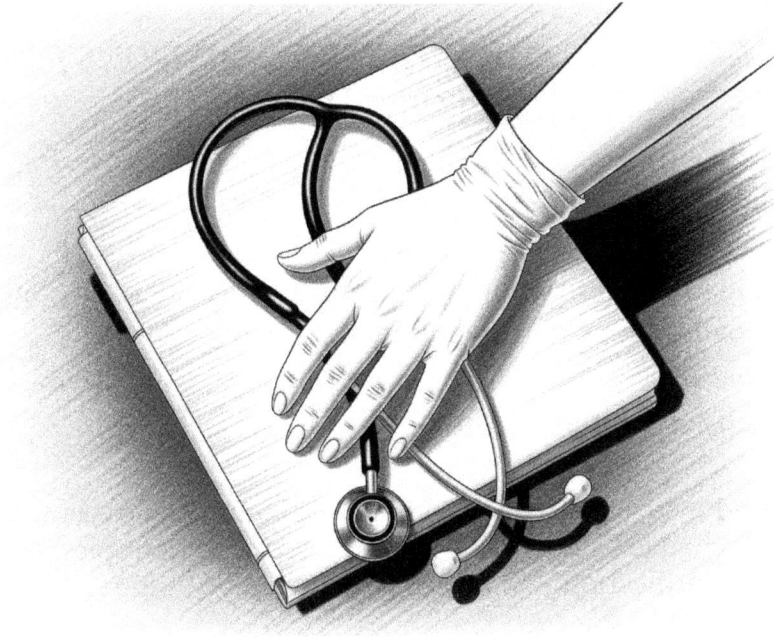

EXERCISE 46. PREPARING QUESTIONS FOR APPOINTMENTS

Objective

Enhance communication with healthcare providers by preparing a list of questions for appointments

Step-by-step instructions

- Review your symptom journal and any recent health changes to identify areas of concern or topics needing clarification.

- Prioritize your questions by importance, focusing on issues that impact your daily life or require immediate attention.

- Write down each question clearly and concisely, ensuring they are specific and relevant to your condition.

- Include questions about medication side effects, lifestyle changes, or new treatment options that you are considering.

- Consider asking about long-term management strategies and preventive measures to improve your quality of life.

- Bring your list of questions to your appointment and refer to it during the discussion to ensure all topics are covered.

- Take notes during the appointment to capture the healthcare provider's responses and any additional advice given.

- Review the answers and advice after the appointment to ensure understanding and to plan any necessary follow-up actions.

Common pitfalls

- Forgetting to ask important questions due to lack of preparation
- Asking vague or overly broad questions that may not yield useful information

Progress tracking

- Evaluate the effectiveness of your questions by assessing the clarity and usefulness of the responses received
- Adjust your question preparation process based on feedback and outcomes from previous appointments

EXERCISE 47. PRACTICING ACTIVE LISTENING

Objective

Enhance communication skills by practicing active listening to improve interactions with healthcare providers and support networks

Step-by-step instructions

- Choose a quiet environment to practice active listening, free from distractions such as phones or television.

- Engage in a conversation with a friend or family member about a topic of mutual interest, ideally related to health or wellness.

- Focus entirely on the speaker, maintaining eye contact and nodding occasionally to show engagement.

- Avoid interrupting or planning your response while the other person is speaking. Instead, concentrate on understanding their message.

- After the speaker finishes, summarize what you heard in your own words to confirm understanding. Use phrases like, "What I hear you saying is..."

- Ask open-ended questions to encourage further discussion and demonstrate interest, such as "Can you tell me more about that?"

- Reflect on the conversation afterward, considering how active listening affected the interaction and what you learned.

- Practice this exercise regularly in different settings, including during healthcare appointments, to strengthen your listening skills.

Common pitfalls

- Allowing distractions to interfere with focus
- Interrupting the speaker or finishing their sentences

Progress tracking

- Keep a journal of your active listening experiences, noting improvements and areas for growth
- Seek feedback from conversation partners on your listening skills to identify strengths and weaknesses

EXERCISE 48. ROLE-PLAYING DOCTOR VISITS

Objective

Improve confidence and effectiveness in communicating with healthcare providers through role-playing scenarios

Step-by-step instructions

- Choose a partner to role-play with, such as a friend or family member, who can act as the healthcare provider.

- Prepare a list of common scenarios you might encounter during a doctor visit, such as discussing new symptoms, medication side effects, or lifestyle changes.

- Select one scenario to focus on for the role-play session.

- Begin the role-play by greeting your partner as you would a healthcare provider and briefly explaining the purpose of your visit.

- Present your concerns or questions clearly and concisely, using the list you prepared in previous exercises as a guide.

- Practice active listening by focusing on your partner's responses, asking follow-up questions, and summarizing their advice to ensure understanding.

- Switch roles with your partner to gain perspective on how healthcare providers might perceive patient interactions.

- Reflect on the role-play session, identifying areas where you felt confident and areas needing improvement.

Common pitfalls

- Overlooking the importance of non-verbal communication, such as eye contact and body language
- Failing to ask clarifying questions when unsure about the information provided

Progress tracking

- Keep a journal of role-play experiences, noting improvements in communication skills and areas for further practice
- Seek feedback from your role-play partner on your communication style and effectiveness

EXERCISE 49. UNDERSTANDING MEDICAL TERMINOLOGY

Objective

Enhance understanding of medical terminology to improve communication with healthcare providers and facilitate effective self-management of chronic diseases

Step-by-step instructions

- Gather a list of common medical terms related to diabetes, hypertension, and musculoskeletal issues. Use reliable sources such as medical websites or educational materials provided by healthcare professionals.

- Dedicate 15-20 minutes daily to study these terms. Focus on understanding their meanings, pronunciation, and context in which they are used.

- Create flashcards with the term on one side and its definition and usage on the other. Review these flashcards regularly to reinforce your memory.

- Practice using these terms in sentences or scenarios related to your health condition. This will help you become more comfortable with the vocabulary during medical appointments.

- Engage in discussions with friends or family members about your condition, incorporating the medical terms you have learned. This will boost your confidence in using the terminology in real-life conversations.

- During healthcare visits, actively listen for these terms and ask for clarification if needed. Use your knowledge to ask informed questions and better understand the information provided by your healthcare provider.

Common pitfalls

- Relying solely on online sources without verifying the accuracy of the information
- Overloading yourself with too many terms at once, leading to confusion

Progress tracking

- Keep a journal of new terms learned and their definitions
- Note instances where understanding medical terminology improved communication with healthcare providers

EXERCISE 50. NOTE-TAKING DURING CONSULTATIONS

Objective

Enhance the ability to take effective notes during medical consultations to improve understanding and recall of healthcare advice

Step-by-step instructions

- Prepare a dedicated notebook or digital device for note-taking during consultations. Ensure it is easily accessible and organized by date or topic.

- Before the appointment, list key questions or concerns you want to address. This will help focus your note-taking on relevant information.

- During the consultation, jot down important points such as diagnosis, treatment options, medication instructions, and lifestyle recommendations. Use bullet points or short phrases for clarity.

- Ask for clarification on any terms or instructions you do not understand. Write down the explanations provided by the healthcare professional.

- Note any follow-up appointments, tests, or referrals mentioned during the visit. Include dates and times if scheduled.

- After the appointment, review your notes to ensure they are complete and understandable. Add any additional details or reflections while the information is fresh in your mind.

- Organize your notes by topic or condition for easy reference in the future. Consider using tabs or digital folders for different health issues.

Common pitfalls

- Failing to review and organize notes promptly after the consultation, leading to incomplete or confusing information
- Overloading notes with unnecessary details, making it difficult to find key information later

Progress tracking

- Keep a record of consultations and note-taking experiences, identifying improvements in clarity and completeness over time
- Evaluate how well your notes help in following medical advice and making informed health decisions

EXERCISE 51. DISCUSSING MEDICATION SIDE EFFECTS

Objective

Improve communication with healthcare providers by effectively discussing medication side effects to enhance self-management of chronic diseases

Step-by-step instructions

- Prepare a list of all medications you are currently taking, including over-the-counter drugs and supplements. Note the dosage and frequency for each.

- Research common side effects associated with each medication using reliable sources such as the medication guide provided by your pharmacist or reputable medical websites.

- Identify any side effects you have experienced. Keep a detailed record, noting the frequency, severity, and any patterns or triggers you observe.

- Prior to your healthcare appointment, write down specific questions or concerns about these side effects. Consider asking about alternative medications or strategies to manage side effects.

- During the consultation, clearly communicate your experiences with side effects. Use your notes to ensure you cover all relevant points and ask for clarification on any medical terms or instructions you do not understand.

- Discuss potential adjustments to your medication regimen with your healthcare provider, such as dosage changes or alternative treatments, to minimize side effects while maintaining efficacy.

- After the appointment, review any new instructions or changes to your medication plan. Update your medication list and side effect log accordingly.

Common pitfalls

- Failing to document side effects consistently, leading to incomplete information during consultations
- Hesitating to discuss side effects due to fear of being perceived as non-compliant

Progress tracking

- Maintain a side effect log to track changes over time and identify patterns
- Evaluate how effectively your discussions with healthcare providers lead to improved management of side effects

EXERCISE 52. CLARIFYING TREATMENT PLANS

Objective

Enhance understanding and clarity of treatment plans to improve adherence and self-management of chronic diseases

Step-by-step instructions

- Gather all relevant documents related to your treatment plan, including prescriptions, test results, and any written instructions from healthcare providers.

- Review each document carefully, highlighting or underlining key information such as medication names, dosages, and specific instructions.

- Create a list of any terms or instructions that are unclear or confusing. Use reliable sources to research these terms, or prepare to ask your healthcare provider for clarification.

- Schedule a dedicated time to discuss your treatment plan with your healthcare provider. Bring your list of questions and any documents that need clarification.

- During the discussion, ask your healthcare provider to explain any unclear aspects of your treatment plan. Take notes on their explanations, using bullet points or short phrases for clarity.

- Confirm your understanding by summarizing the key points of your treatment plan back to your healthcare

provider. Ask for confirmation or further clarification if
needed.

- After the discussion, review your notes and update your
treatment plan documents with any new information or
changes. Ensure all instructions are clear and complete.

Common pitfalls

- Neglecting to ask for clarification on confusing terms or
instructions, leading to misunderstandings
- Failing to update treatment plan documents with new
information, resulting in outdated or incorrect guidance

Progress tracking

- Keep a record of treatment plan discussions and note any
improvements in understanding and adherence over time
- Evaluate how well your clarified treatment plan supports
effective self-management and symptom reduction

EXERCISE 53. EXPRESSING CONCERNS CLEARLY

Objective

Enhance the ability to express health concerns clearly to healthcare providers for improved chronic disease management

Step-by-step instructions

- Identify specific concerns related to your chronic condition, such as symptoms, treatment side effects, or lifestyle challenges. Write them down in a clear and concise manner.

- Prioritize your concerns by ranking them based on urgency or impact on your daily life. Focus on the top three to discuss during your healthcare appointment.

- Use descriptive language to articulate your concerns. Include details such as frequency, duration, and intensity of symptoms or issues.

- Practice expressing your concerns aloud, either alone or with a trusted friend or family member, to build confidence and clarity in your communication.

- Prepare a list of questions related to your concerns. Consider asking about potential causes, treatment options, or lifestyle adjustments that could address your issues.

- During your appointment, clearly state your top concerns at the beginning of the conversation. Use your notes to ensure you cover all relevant points.

- Ask for clarification on any responses or recommendations from your healthcare provider that you do not fully understand. Take notes on their explanations for future reference.

Common pitfalls

- Overloading the conversation with too many concerns, leading to a lack of focus
- Using vague or non-specific language, which can hinder effective communication

Progress tracking

- Keep a record of each healthcare appointment, noting how well your concerns were addressed
- Evaluate any improvements in symptom management or treatment outcomes following discussions with your healthcare provider

EXERCISE 54. BUILDING A SUPPORT NETWORK

Objective

Develop a reliable support network to enhance self-management of chronic diseases

Step-by-step instructions

- Identify key individuals in your life who can provide support, such as family members, friends, or colleagues. Consider their availability, willingness, and ability to assist you.

- Reach out to these individuals and discuss your chronic condition, explaining how they can help you manage it. Be specific about the type of support you need, such as emotional encouragement, assistance with daily tasks, or accountability for lifestyle changes.

- Explore local or online support groups related to your condition. These groups can offer shared experiences, advice, and emotional support from others facing similar challenges.

- Schedule regular check-ins with your support network, whether in person, by phone, or through video calls. Use these opportunities to share updates on your condition, discuss any challenges, and seek advice or encouragement.

- Encourage open communication within your support network. Let them know how they can best support you and be receptive to their feedback or suggestions.

- Consider involving a healthcare professional, such as a counselor or therapist, to provide additional support and guidance. They can offer strategies for coping with stress and managing your condition effectively.

- Evaluate the effectiveness of your support network periodically. Reflect on whether your needs are being met and make adjustments as necessary, such as adding new members or seeking different types of support.

Common pitfalls

- Relying too heavily on a single individual, which can lead to burnout or strained relationships
- Failing to communicate your needs clearly, resulting in misunderstandings or inadequate support

Progress tracking

- Keep a journal of interactions with your support network, noting any positive impacts on your condition management
- Assess changes in your ability to manage symptoms and adhere to treatment plans with the help of your support network

EXERCISE 55. FOLLOWING UP ON APPOINTMENTS

Objective

Ensure effective follow-up on healthcare appointments to enhance chronic disease management

Step-by-step instructions

- Schedule your next appointment before leaving the current one. Confirm the date and time, and set a reminder on your phone or calendar.

- Request a summary of the visit from your healthcare provider, including any changes in treatment plans, new prescriptions, or recommended lifestyle adjustments.

- Review the visit summary at home. Note any questions or concerns that arise and add them to your list for the next appointment.

- Follow through on any prescribed actions, such as filling prescriptions, scheduling tests, or making lifestyle changes. Keep a record of your progress and any challenges you encounter.

- If you experience new symptoms or side effects, document them with details such as onset, frequency, and severity. This information will be valuable for your next appointment.

- Contact your healthcare provider if you have urgent questions or if your condition worsens before your next scheduled visit. Use the contact information provided during your appointment.

- Prepare for your next appointment by reviewing your notes, progress, and any new concerns. Bring all relevant documents, such as test results or medication lists, to the appointment.

Common pitfalls

- Forgetting to schedule follow-up appointments, leading to gaps in care
- Neglecting to document symptoms or changes, which can hinder effective treatment adjustments

Progress tracking

- Maintain a log of appointments, including dates, key discussions, and outcomes
- Evaluate improvements in symptom management and overall health following each appointment

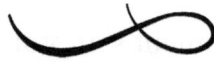

Chapter 16: Reading Food Labels Exercise

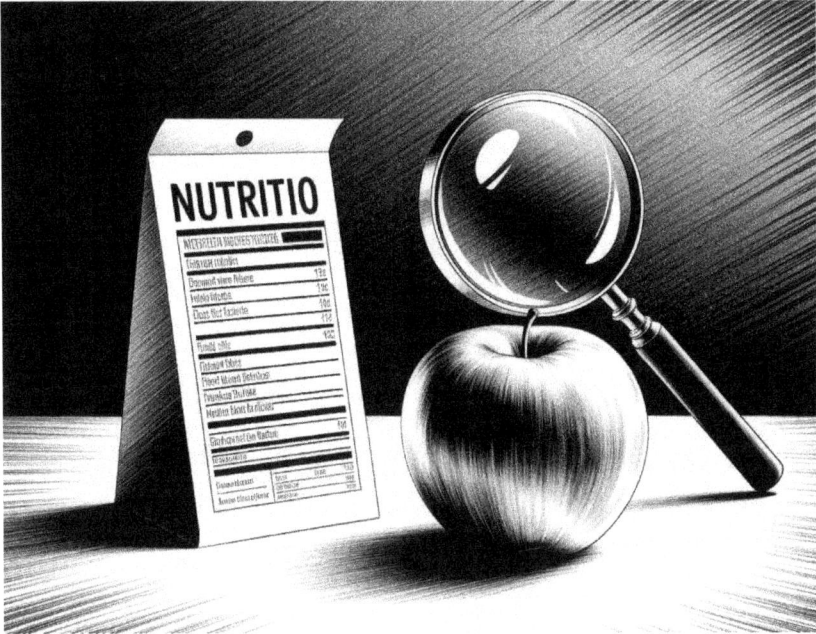

EXERCISE 56. UNDERSTANDING SERVING SIZES

Objective

Gain a clear understanding of serving sizes to better manage dietary intake and support chronic disease management

Step-by-step instructions

- Familiarize yourself with the concept of serving sizes by reviewing the nutrition facts label on packaged foods. Note the serving size listed and the number of servings per container.

- Use measuring cups, spoons, or a food scale to accurately measure out a single serving according to the label. This will help you visualize what a standard serving looks like.

- Compare the measured serving size to the portion you typically consume. Adjust your portion sizes if necessary to align with recommended serving sizes for better dietary control.

- Practice estimating serving sizes for common foods without measuring tools. For example, a serving of meat is roughly the size of a deck of cards, and a serving of cooked pasta is about the size of a baseball.

- Keep a food diary to track your daily intake, noting the number of servings consumed for each food item. This will help you identify patterns and make adjustments to your diet as needed.

- Educate yourself on the recommended daily servings for different food groups based on dietary guidelines. Use this information to plan balanced meals that support your health goals.

- Be mindful of serving sizes when dining out. Restaurants often serve larger portions, so consider sharing a dish or taking half home to maintain appropriate serving sizes.

Common pitfalls

- Confusing portion size with serving size, leading to unintentional overeating
- Neglecting to adjust serving sizes for high-calorie or high-sodium foods, which can impact chronic disease management

Progress tracking

- Regularly review your food diary to assess adherence to serving size recommendations
- Monitor changes in weight, blood sugar levels, or blood pressure as indicators of improved dietary management

EXERCISE 57. IDENTIFYING ADDED SUGARS

Objective

Identify and reduce the intake of added sugars to support chronic disease management

Step-by-step instructions

- Familiarize yourself with common names for added sugars, such as high fructose corn syrup, cane sugar, and dextrose. This will help you recognize them on ingredient lists.

- Examine the nutrition facts label on packaged foods. Look for the "Added Sugars" line under "Total Sugars" to determine how much sugar has been added.

- Compare the amount of added sugars to the recommended daily limit. The American Heart Association suggests no more than 36 grams (9 teaspoons) for men and 25 grams (6 teaspoons) for women per day.

- Identify foods and beverages in your diet that are high in added sugars, such as sodas, candies, and baked goods. Consider healthier alternatives or reducing portion sizes.

- Keep a daily log of your sugar intake, noting the sources and amounts of added sugars consumed. This will help you track your progress and make necessary adjustments.

- Gradually reduce your consumption of added sugars by making small changes, such as choosing unsweetened versions of products or using natural sweeteners like fruit.

- Educate yourself on the health impacts of excessive sugar intake, including its role in diabetes, hypertension, and musculoskeletal issues, to reinforce your motivation for change.

Common pitfalls

- Overlooking hidden sugars in processed foods, leading to unintentional overconsumption
- Relying on "sugar-free" products that may contain other unhealthy additives

Progress tracking

- Regularly review your sugar intake log to assess adherence to recommended limits
- Monitor changes in blood sugar levels, blood pressure, or weight as indicators of improved dietary management

EXERCISE 58. RECOGNIZING WHOLE GRAINS

Objective

Identify and incorporate whole grains into your diet to support
chronic disease management

Step-by-step instructions

- Familiarize yourself with common whole grains such as
  brown rice, quinoa, oats, barley, and whole wheat. These
  grains retain all parts of the grain kernel, providing more
  nutrients and fiber.

- Examine food labels for the term "whole grain" or
  "whole" before the grain name in the ingredient list.
  Ensure that whole grains are listed as one of the first
  ingredients to confirm they are a primary component.

- Compare products by checking the fiber content on the
  nutrition facts label. Whole grain products typically have
  higher fiber content, which is beneficial for managing
  blood sugar levels and promoting heart health.

- Identify refined grains in your diet, such as white bread,
  white rice, and regular pasta. Gradually replace these
  with whole grain alternatives to improve nutritional
  intake.

- Keep a daily log of your grain consumption, noting the
  types and amounts of whole grains consumed. This will
  help you track your progress and make necessary
  adjustments.

- Experiment with incorporating whole grains into your meals, such as using whole wheat bread for sandwiches, adding quinoa to salads, or choosing oatmeal for breakfast.

- Educate yourself on the health benefits of whole grains, including their role in reducing the risk of diabetes, hypertension, and musculoskeletal issues, to reinforce your motivation for change.

Common pitfalls

- Confusing "multigrain" or "stone-ground" with whole grain, which may not provide the same nutritional benefits
- Overlooking the importance of portion control, even with whole grains, to maintain balanced dietary intake

Progress tracking

- Regularly review your grain consumption log to assess adherence to whole grain recommendations
- Monitor changes in blood sugar levels, blood pressure, or digestive health as indicators of improved dietary management

EXERCISE 59. SPOTTING TRANS FATS

Objective

Identify and reduce the intake of trans fats to support chronic
disease management

Step-by-step instructions

- Familiarize yourself with common sources of trans fats,
  such as partially hydrogenated oils, which are often found
  in processed foods like baked goods, snacks, and fried
  items.

- Examine the nutrition facts label on packaged foods.
  Look for the "Trans Fat" line under "Total Fat" to
  determine the amount present. Aim for products with 0
  grams of trans fat.

- Check the ingredient list for terms like "partially
  hydrogenated" or "hydrogenated" oils, which indicate the
  presence of trans fats, even if the label states 0 grams.
  Products can contain up to 0.5 grams per serving and still
  be labeled as 0 grams.

- Identify foods in your diet that are high in trans fats, such
  as margarine, shortening, and certain packaged snacks.
  Consider healthier alternatives or reducing portion sizes.

- Keep a daily log of your trans fat intake, noting the
  sources and amounts consumed. This will help you track
  your progress and make necessary adjustments.

- Gradually reduce your consumption of trans fats by making small changes, such as choosing products labeled "trans fat-free" or using healthier fats like olive oil.

- Educate yourself on the health impacts of trans fats, including their role in increasing the risk of heart disease, diabetes, and hypertension, to reinforce your motivation for change

Common pitfalls

- Overlooking small amounts of trans fats in multiple servings, leading to unintentional overconsumption
- Assuming "cholesterol-free" or "low-fat" products are also free of trans fats

Progress tracking

- Regularly review your trans fat intake log to assess adherence to recommended limits
- Monitor changes in cholesterol levels, blood pressure, or weight as indicators of improved dietary management

EXERCISE 60. SODIUM CONTENT AWARENESS

Objective

Increase awareness of sodium content in foods to support chronic disease management

Step-by-step instructions

- Familiarize yourself with the recommended daily sodium intake, which is less than 2,300 milligrams for most adults, and ideally around 1,500 milligrams for those with hypertension or diabetes.

- Examine the nutrition facts label on packaged foods. Look for the "Sodium" line to determine the amount per serving. Aim for products with lower sodium content.

- Check the ingredient list for terms like "sodium," "salt," "sodium chloride," "monosodium glutamate (MSG)," and "baking soda," which indicate the presence of sodium.

- Identify high-sodium foods in your diet, such as processed meats, canned soups, and salty snacks. Consider healthier alternatives or reducing portion sizes.

- Keep a daily log of your sodium intake, noting the sources and amounts consumed. This will help you track your progress and make necessary adjustments.

- Gradually reduce your consumption of high-sodium foods by making small changes, such as choosing fresh or frozen vegetables over canned ones, and using herbs and spices instead of salt for flavor.

- Educate yourself on the health impacts of excessive sodium intake, including its role in increasing the risk of hypertension, heart disease, and kidney issues, to reinforce your motivation for change

Common pitfalls

- Overlooking sodium content in condiments and sauces, which can significantly contribute to daily intake
- Assuming "low-fat" or "healthy" labeled products are also low in sodium

Progress tracking

- Regularly review your sodium intake log to assess adherence to recommended limits
- Monitor changes in blood pressure or fluid retention as indicators of improved dietary management

EXERCISE 61. FIBER CONTENT EVALUATION

Objective

Increase awareness of fiber content in foods to support chronic
disease management

Step-by-step instructions

- Familiarize yourself with the recommended daily fiber
  intake, which is 25 grams for women and 38 grams for
  men, or 14 grams per 1,000 calories consumed.

- Examine the nutrition facts label on packaged foods.
  Look for the "Dietary Fiber" line under "Total
  Carbohydrate" to determine the amount per serving. Aim
  for products with higher fiber content.

- Check the ingredient list for terms like "whole grain,"
  "whole wheat," "bran," and "fiber," which indicate the
  presence of dietary fiber.

- Identify low-fiber foods in your diet, such as white bread,
  white rice, and processed snacks. Consider healthier
  alternatives like whole grain bread, brown rice, and fresh
  fruits and vegetables.

- Keep a daily log of your fiber intake, noting the sources
  and amounts consumed. This will help you track your
  progress and make necessary adjustments.

- Gradually increase your consumption of high-fiber foods by making small changes, such as adding a serving of vegetables to each meal or choosing whole grain options.

- Educate yourself on the health benefits of fiber, including its role in improving digestion, controlling blood sugar levels, and reducing the risk of heart disease, to reinforce your motivation for change

Common pitfalls

- Overlooking fiber content in processed foods, which can be misleading due to added fibers
- Assuming "whole grain" or "multigrain" labels always indicate high fiber content

Progress tracking

- Regularly review your fiber intake log to assess adherence to recommended levels
- Monitor changes in digestion, blood sugar levels, or cholesterol as indicators of improved dietary management

EXERCISE 62. INTERPRETING INGREDIENT LISTS

Objective

Enhance understanding of ingredient lists to make informed dietary choices for chronic disease management

Step-by-step instructions

- Familiarize yourself with common ingredient list terms, such as "sugar," "sucrose," "high fructose corn syrup," "partially hydrogenated oils," and "enriched flour," which can indicate added sugars, unhealthy fats, and refined grains.

- Identify the order of ingredients, noting that they are listed by weight from highest to lowest. Focus on the first three ingredients as they make up the majority of the product.

- Look for whole food ingredients, such as "whole grain," "oats," "brown rice," "quinoa," and "nuts," which are beneficial for managing diabetes, hypertension, and musculoskeletal issues.

- Be cautious of long ingredient lists, which often indicate highly processed foods. Aim for products with fewer, recognizable ingredients.

- Recognize artificial additives and preservatives, such as "aspartame," "sodium benzoate," and "artificial flavors," which may not support optimal health.

- Keep a log of products you frequently purchase, noting their ingredient lists. This will help you identify patterns and make healthier choices over time.

- Educate yourself on the impact of certain ingredients on chronic diseases, such as the role of added sugars in blood sugar spikes or the effect of trans fats on heart health, to reinforce your motivation for change

Common pitfalls

- Assuming "natural" or "organic" labels mean the product is free of unhealthy ingredients
- Overlooking the presence of multiple forms of sugar or fat listed separately in the ingredients

Progress tracking

- Regularly review your ingredient list log to assess improvements in your food choices
- Monitor changes in symptoms or overall health as indicators of better dietary management

EXERCISE 63. DETECTING ARTIFICIAL ADDITIVES

Objective

Enhance the ability to identify artificial additives in food products to support chronic disease management

Step-by-step instructions

- Familiarize yourself with common artificial additives, such as "aspartame," "monosodium glutamate (MSG)," "sodium benzoate," "artificial flavors," and "artificial colors" like "Red 40" or "Yellow 5."

- Examine the ingredient list on food packaging. Look for any of the identified artificial additives, which are often listed towards the end of the ingredient list.

- Identify products with long ingredient lists, as these are more likely to contain artificial additives. Aim for foods with fewer, recognizable ingredients.

- Be cautious of terms like "flavoring" or "coloring," which can indicate the presence of artificial substances. Seek out products that specify "natural flavors" or "natural colors."

- Keep a log of products you frequently purchase, noting the presence of artificial additives. This will help you identify patterns and make healthier choices over time.

- Educate yourself on the potential health impacts of artificial additives, such as their role in exacerbating symptoms of chronic diseases, to reinforce your motivation for change

Common pitfalls

- Assuming "natural" or "organic" labels mean the product is free of artificial additives
- Overlooking the presence of multiple artificial additives listed separately in the ingredients

Progress tracking

- Regularly review your additive log to assess improvements in your food choices
- Monitor changes in symptoms or overall health as indicators of better dietary management

EXERCISE 64. COMPARING NUTRITIONAL VALUES

Objective

Enhance the ability to compare nutritional values to make informed dietary choices for chronic disease management

Step-by-step instructions

- Select two similar food products, such as two brands of cereal or two types of bread, to compare their nutritional labels.

- Examine the serving size on each product's label to ensure you are comparing equivalent portions.

- Compare the total calories per serving, noting which product offers fewer calories if weight management is a concern.

- Look at the total carbohydrates, focusing on the amount of dietary fiber and sugars. Choose products with higher fiber and lower sugar content to better manage blood sugar levels.

- Check the total fat content, paying attention to saturated and trans fats. Opt for products with lower amounts of these unhealthy fats to support heart health.

- Review the sodium content, especially if managing hypertension. Select products with lower sodium levels to help maintain healthy blood pressure.

- Consider the protein content, as higher protein can aid in muscle maintenance and satiety.

- Note any vitamins and minerals listed, such as calcium, iron, or vitamin D, which can contribute to overall health and support musculoskeletal function.

- Keep a log of your comparisons to track which products consistently offer better nutritional profiles.

Common pitfalls

- Focusing solely on calorie count without considering nutrient quality
- Ignoring serving size differences, leading to inaccurate comparisons

Progress tracking

- Regularly update your log with new product comparisons to refine your choices
- Monitor changes in symptoms or overall health as indicators of improved dietary management

EXERCISE 65. ALLERGEN IDENTIFICATION

Objective

Improve the ability to identify potential allergens in food products to support chronic disease management

Step-by-step instructions

- Familiarize yourself with common allergens, such as "peanuts," "tree nuts," "milk," "eggs," "wheat," "soy," "fish," and "shellfish."

- Examine the ingredient list on food packaging. Look for any of the identified allergens, which are often highlighted in bold or listed separately under a "Contains" statement.

- Be aware of cross-contamination warnings, such as "may contain" or "processed in a facility that also processes," which indicate potential exposure to allergens.

- Identify products with vague ingredient descriptions like "spices" or "natural flavors," which can sometimes include allergens. Contact the manufacturer if clarification is needed.

- Keep a log of products you frequently purchase, noting the presence of allergens. This will help you identify patterns and make safer choices over time.

- Educate yourself on the potential health impacts of allergens, such as their role in exacerbating symptoms of chronic diseases, to reinforce your motivation for change

Common pitfalls

- Assuming "gluten-free" labels mean the product is free of all allergens
- Overlooking the presence of allergens in non-food items like supplements or medications

Progress tracking

- Regularly review your allergen log to assess improvements in your food choices
- Monitor changes in symptoms or overall health as indicators of better allergen management

EXERCISE 66. CALORIE COUNTING BASICS

Objective

Understand the basics of calorie counting to support effective self-management of chronic diseases

Step-by-step instructions

- Determine your daily calorie needs using an online calculator or consult with a healthcare professional to get a personalized recommendation based on your age, gender, weight, height, and activity level.

- Keep a food diary for at least one week, recording everything you eat and drink, including portion sizes. Use a digital app or a notebook for convenience.

- Use a reliable calorie counting app or website to look up the calorie content of each item in your food diary. Pay attention to portion sizes to ensure accuracy.

- Calculate the total calories consumed each day by adding up the calories from all food and drink items recorded in your diary.

- Compare your daily calorie intake to your recommended daily calorie needs. Identify any patterns or discrepancies that may be affecting your chronic disease management.

- Adjust your portion sizes or food choices to better align with your calorie needs, focusing on nutrient-dense foods that support overall health.

- Monitor your progress by regularly updating your food diary and calorie calculations, making adjustments as needed to maintain or achieve your health goals.

Common pitfalls

- Underestimating portion sizes, leading to inaccurate calorie counts
- Ignoring the calorie content of beverages, which can contribute significantly to daily intake

Progress tracking

- Review your food diary weekly to assess adherence to your calorie goals
- Track changes in weight, energy levels, and symptoms to evaluate the impact of calorie management on your chronic disease control

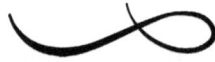

Chapter 17: Managing Medication Schedules and Exercise

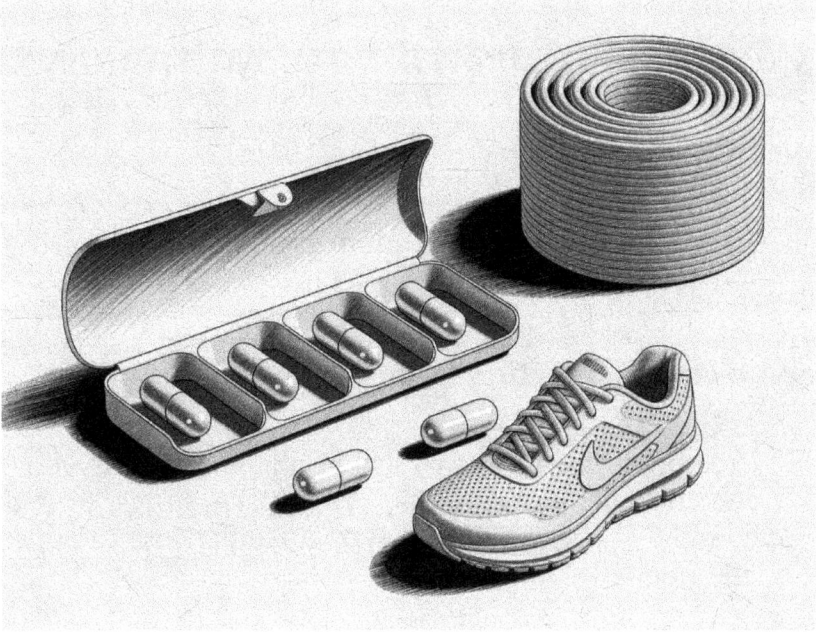

EXERCISE 67. MEDICATION TIMING AWARENESS

Objective

Enhance awareness of medication timing to optimize the
effectiveness of treatment for chronic diseases

Step-by-step instructions

- Create a comprehensive list of all medications you are
  currently taking, including prescription drugs, over-the-
  counter medications, and supplements. Note the dosage
  and frequency for each.

- Consult with your healthcare provider or pharmacist to
  confirm the optimal timing for each medication. Consider
  factors such as food interactions, time of day, and other
  medications.

- Develop a daily medication schedule that incorporates
  the recommended timing for each medication. Use a
  digital app, calendar, or a written planner to organize
  your schedule.

- Set reminders or alarms on your phone or other devices
  to alert you when it's time to take each medication.
  Ensure the reminders are set for the correct times based
  on your schedule.

- Monitor your adherence to the medication schedule by
  keeping a log of when you take each dose. Note any
  missed doses and the reasons for them.

- Review your medication log regularly to identify patterns or challenges in maintaining your schedule. Adjust your reminders or schedule as needed to improve adherence.

- Communicate any difficulties or side effects with your healthcare provider to explore potential adjustments to your medication regimen.

Common pitfalls

- Forgetting to adjust medication timing when traveling across time zones
- Overlooking the impact of dietary changes on medication absorption

Progress tracking

- Track your adherence to the medication schedule by reviewing your log weekly
- Monitor changes in symptoms or overall health to assess the effectiveness of your medication timing adjustments

EXERCISE 68. PILL ORGANIZER SETUP

Objective

Organize medications effectively to ensure consistent and accurate dosing for chronic disease management

Step-by-step instructions

- Gather all medications, including prescription drugs, over-the-counter medications, and supplements. Ensure you have enough supply for at least one week.

- Obtain a pill organizer with compartments for each day of the week and, if needed, multiple times per day (morning, afternoon, evening, bedtime).

- Review your medication list, noting the dosage and frequency for each. Confirm this information with your healthcare provider or pharmacist if necessary.

- Allocate a specific time each week to set up your pill organizer, such as Sunday evening. Make this a routine to ensure consistency.

- Fill each compartment of the pill organizer according to your medication schedule. Double-check each compartment to ensure accuracy.

- Store the pill organizer in a visible, easily accessible location to remind you to take your medications as scheduled.

- Set daily reminders on your phone or other devices to prompt you to take your medications at the designated times.

- Monitor your adherence by keeping a log of when you take each dose. Note any missed doses and the reasons for them.

Common pitfalls

- Forgetting to refill the pill organizer weekly, leading to missed doses
- Mixing up medications when filling the organizer, resulting in incorrect dosing

Progress tracking

- Review your medication log weekly to assess adherence and identify any patterns of missed doses
- Track changes in symptoms or overall health to evaluate the impact of consistent medication management

EXERCISE 69. SETTING MEDICATION REMINDERS

Objective

Ensure timely medication intake to enhance treatment effectiveness and support chronic disease management

Step-by-step instructions

- Identify all medications you need to take, including prescription drugs, over-the-counter medications, and supplements. Note the specific times each should be taken.

- Choose a reliable method for setting reminders, such as a smartphone app, digital calendar, or alarm clock. Ensure the method is easily accessible and suits your daily routine.

- Program reminders for each medication dose, specifying the exact time and any necessary instructions (e.g., take with food, avoid certain activities).

- Test the reminder system for a few days to ensure it functions correctly and fits seamlessly into your daily schedule.

- Adjust reminder settings as needed to accommodate changes in your routine, such as travel or schedule shifts.

- Keep a backup reminder system, like a written schedule or a secondary device, in case of technical issues with your primary method.

- Regularly review and update your reminder system to reflect any changes in your medication regimen or lifestyle.

Common pitfalls

- Ignoring reminders due to busy schedules or distractions
- Failing to update reminders when medication regimens change

Progress tracking

- Monitor your adherence by noting any missed doses and the reasons for them
- Evaluate the effectiveness of your reminder system by tracking changes in symptoms or overall health

EXERCISE 70. UNDERSTANDING MEDICATION LABELS

Objective

Enhance understanding of medication labels to ensure safe and effective use of medications for chronic disease management

Step-by-step instructions

- Gather all medications, including prescription drugs, over-the-counter medications, and supplements. Have a notepad or digital device ready for notes.

- Examine each medication label carefully. Identify key information such as the medication name, dosage, frequency, and any special instructions (e.g., take with food, avoid alcohol).

- Note the expiration date on each label. Ensure that all medications are within their expiration period to maintain effectiveness and safety.

- Look for any warnings or contraindications on the label. These may include potential side effects, interactions with other medications, or conditions that may be affected by the medication.

- If any information is unclear or missing, consult your healthcare provider or pharmacist for clarification. Do not make assumptions about medication use.

- Create a medication chart or list that includes all relevant information from the labels. This should include the medication name, dosage, frequency, special instructions, and expiration date.

- Store medications in their original containers to preserve label information and prevent mix-ups. Keep them in a cool, dry place away from direct sunlight.

- Regularly review and update your medication chart or list, especially when there are changes in your medication regimen or new prescriptions are added.

Common pitfalls

- Misinterpreting label instructions, leading to incorrect dosing
- Overlooking expiration dates, resulting in the use of ineffective or unsafe medications

Progress tracking

- Periodically review your medication chart to ensure all information is current and accurate
- Track any changes in symptoms or side effects to assess the impact of medication adherence and understanding

EXERCISE 71. TRACKING MEDICATION SIDE EFFECTS

Objective

Identify and manage side effects of medications to enhance treatment safety and effectiveness

Step-by-step instructions

- Gather all medications, including prescription drugs, over-the-counter medications, and supplements. Have a notepad or digital device ready for notes.

- Review the information provided with each medication, focusing on the section detailing potential side effects. Note any side effects that are common or serious.

- Create a side effect tracking chart. Include columns for the date, time, medication taken, observed side effects, severity, and any actions taken (e.g., contacting a healthcare provider).

- Monitor your body's reactions after taking each medication. Record any side effects in your chart, noting the time they occur and their intensity.

- If you experience a new or worsening side effect, consult your healthcare provider promptly. Provide them with your tracking chart for a detailed overview.

- Adjust your medication regimen only under the guidance of a healthcare professional. Do not stop or change medications without consulting them first.

- Regularly review your side effect tracking chart to identify patterns or trends. Use this information to discuss potential adjustments with your healthcare provider.

Common pitfalls

- Overlooking mild side effects that could indicate a developing issue
- Failing to record side effects consistently, leading to incomplete information for healthcare providers

Progress tracking

- Evaluate the frequency and severity of side effects over time to assess the impact of medication adjustments
- Track any changes in overall health or symptoms to determine the effectiveness of side effect management

EXERCISE 72. COMMUNICATING WITH PHARMACISTS

Objective

Enhance communication skills with pharmacists to optimize medication management and ensure safe, effective treatment for chronic diseases

Step-by-step instructions

- Prepare a list of all current medications, including prescription drugs, over-the-counter medications, and supplements. Include the name, dosage, frequency, and any known side effects.

- Identify any specific questions or concerns you have about your medications. These might include potential side effects, interactions with other drugs, or alternative options.

- Visit your pharmacy during a less busy time to ensure the pharmacist can give you adequate attention. Early mornings or mid-afternoons are often quieter.

- Introduce yourself to the pharmacist and briefly explain your chronic conditions. This context can help them provide more tailored advice.

- Present your medication list and questions to the pharmacist. Be clear and concise in your communication to ensure all concerns are addressed.

- Take notes during the conversation. Record any important information or recommendations provided by the pharmacist.

- Ask for clarification if any information is unclear. Do not hesitate to request further explanation or examples to ensure full understanding.

- Inquire about any available resources or services the pharmacy offers, such as medication synchronization or automatic refills, to help manage your medication schedule.

- Thank the pharmacist for their assistance and confirm any follow-up actions you need to take, such as scheduling a medication review or contacting your healthcare provider.

Common pitfalls

- Failing to prepare a comprehensive medication list, leading to incomplete information for the pharmacist
- Not asking for clarification on complex medical terms or instructions

Progress tracking

- Keep a record of all pharmacist interactions, noting any changes in medication or advice given
- Monitor any improvements in medication adherence or symptom management following pharmacist consultations

EXERCISE 73. REVIEWING MEDICATION INTERACTIONS

Objective

Understand and manage potential interactions between medications to ensure safe and effective treatment for chronic diseases

Step-by-step instructions

- Collect all medications, including prescription drugs, over-the-counter medications, and supplements. Have a notepad or digital device ready for notes.

- Review the information provided with each medication, focusing on the section detailing potential drug interactions. Note any interactions that are common or serious.

- Create a medication interaction chart. Include columns for the medication name, potential interactions, observed effects, and any actions taken (e.g., consulting a healthcare provider).

- Use a reliable online drug interaction checker or consult a pharmacist to identify any potential interactions between your medications. Record any findings in your chart.

- Monitor your body's reactions when taking medications together. Record any unusual symptoms or changes in your chart, noting the time they occur and their intensity.

- If you suspect a medication interaction, consult your healthcare provider promptly. Provide them with your interaction chart for a detailed overview.

- Adjust your medication regimen only under the guidance of a healthcare professional. Do not stop or change medications without consulting them first.

- Regularly review your medication interaction chart to identify patterns or trends. Use this information to discuss potential adjustments with your healthcare provider.

Common pitfalls

- Overlooking interactions with over-the-counter medications or supplements
- Failing to record interactions consistently, leading to incomplete information for healthcare providers

Progress tracking

- Evaluate the frequency and severity of interactions over time to assess the impact of medication adjustments
- Track any changes in overall health or symptoms to determine the effectiveness of interaction management

EXERCISE 74. CREATING A MEDICATION LOG

Objective

Develop a comprehensive medication log to enhance medication
adherence and ensure effective management of chronic diseases

Step-by-step instructions

- Gather all current medications, including prescription
  drugs, over-the-counter medications, and supplements.
  Ensure you have the name, dosage, frequency, and any
  special instructions for each.

- Choose a format for your medication log. This could be a
  notebook, a digital spreadsheet, or a medication
  management app. Select a format that is convenient and
  easy for you to update regularly.

- Create columns in your log for the following information:
  medication name, dosage, frequency, time of day to take,
  and any special instructions or notes (e.g., take with
  food).

- Enter each medication into your log, filling out all
  relevant columns. Double-check the information for
  accuracy to prevent any errors in your medication
  schedule.

- Set reminders for each medication dose. Use alarms on
  your phone, a digital calendar, or a medication
  management app to alert you when it's time to take your
  medication.

- Update your log regularly. Whenever there is a change in your medication regimen, such as a new prescription or a dosage adjustment, promptly update your log to reflect these changes.

- Review your medication log weekly. Check for any missed doses or inconsistencies and make necessary adjustments to improve adherence.

- Share your medication log with your healthcare provider during appointments. This will help them understand your current regimen and make informed decisions about your treatment plan.

Common pitfalls

- Forgetting to update the log with new medications or dosage changes
- Not setting reminders, leading to missed doses

Progress tracking

- Monitor adherence by noting any missed doses and identifying patterns or reasons for non-adherence
- Evaluate the impact of consistent medication adherence on symptom management and overall health improvement

EXERCISE 75. ADJUSTING MEDICATION TIMING

Objective

Optimize medication timing to enhance effectiveness and minimize side effects

Step-by-step instructions

- Gather all medications, including prescription drugs, over-the-counter medications, and supplements. Have a notepad or digital device ready for notes.

- Review the instructions for each medication, focusing on the recommended timing and any specific requirements (e.g., take with food, avoid certain times of day).

- Create a daily medication schedule. Include columns for medication name, dosage, recommended time, and any special instructions.

- Consider your daily routine and identify optimal times for taking each medication. Ensure these times align with the medication's requirements and your lifestyle.

- Set reminders for each medication dose. Use alarms on your phone, a digital calendar, or a medication management app to alert you when it's time to take your medication.

- Monitor your body's reactions to the adjusted timing. Record any changes in symptoms, side effects, or overall well-being in your notes.

- Consult your healthcare provider to discuss any significant changes in your medication timing. Provide them with your schedule and observations for a detailed overview.

- Adjust your medication timing only under the guidance of a healthcare professional. Do not make changes without consulting them first.

Common pitfalls

- Ignoring specific timing instructions, leading to reduced medication effectiveness
- Failing to consider lifestyle factors, resulting in missed doses or inconsistent timing

Progress tracking

- Evaluate the impact of timing adjustments on symptom management and overall health
- Track any changes in side effects or medication effectiveness to determine the success of timing modifications

EXERCISE 76. MANAGING MISSED DOSES

Objective

Develop strategies to effectively manage missed medication doses and minimize their impact on chronic disease management

Step-by-step instructions

- Identify the missed dose as soon as possible. Check your medication log or reminders to confirm the missed dose.

- Refer to the medication's instructions or consult your healthcare provider to determine the appropriate action for a missed dose. Some medications may require taking the missed dose immediately, while others may advise skipping it.

- If instructed to take the missed dose, do so as soon as you remember, unless it is close to the time of your next scheduled dose. In that case, skip the missed dose and resume your regular schedule.

- Avoid doubling up on doses to make up for a missed one, unless specifically directed by your healthcare provider.

- Record the missed dose in your medication log, noting the date, time, and any actions taken. This will help you track patterns and discuss them with your healthcare provider.

- Set up additional reminders or alarms to prevent future missed doses. Consider using a medication management app with customizable alerts.

- Discuss any recurring issues with missed doses with your healthcare provider. They may suggest adjustments to your medication regimen or offer additional strategies to improve adherence.

Common pitfalls

- Taking a missed dose too close to the next scheduled dose, leading to potential overdose
- Failing to consult healthcare providers for guidance on handling missed doses

Progress tracking

- Monitor the frequency of missed doses and identify any patterns or triggers
- Evaluate the impact of improved adherence on symptom control and overall health

EXERCISE 77. UNDERSTANDING PRESCRIPTION REFILLS

Objective

Gain a clear understanding of how to manage prescription refills
effectively to ensure continuous medication adherence

Step-by-step instructions

- Identify all medications that require regular refills. Make
  a list including the medication name, dosage, and refill
  frequency.

- Check the prescription label for the number of refills
  remaining. Note the expiration date of the prescription to
  ensure it is still valid.

- Set a reminder to request a refill at least one week before
  your current supply runs out. Use a digital calendar,
  phone alarm, or medication management app for alerts.

- Contact your pharmacy to request a refill. Confirm the
  pickup or delivery date and time to avoid any delays.

- If your prescription has no refills remaining, contact your
  healthcare provider to request a new prescription. Allow
  sufficient time for processing and approval.

- Keep a record of refill dates and any communication with
  your pharmacy or healthcare provider. This will help

track your medication supply and identify any potential issues.

- Discuss any difficulties with refills, such as insurance coverage or pharmacy availability, with your healthcare provider. They may offer alternative solutions or assistance.

Common pitfalls

- Waiting until the last minute to request a refill, leading to missed doses
- Overlooking the prescription expiration date, resulting in delays

Progress tracking

- Monitor the consistency of your medication supply and identify any patterns of delay
- Evaluate the impact of timely refills on symptom management and overall health

EXERCISE 78. SAFE MEDICATION DISPOSAL

Objective

Ensure safe and environmentally responsible disposal of unused or expired medications to prevent accidental ingestion and environmental contamination

Step-by-step instructions

- Review your medication inventory regularly, at least every three months, to identify any expired or unused medications.

- Check the medication label or patient information leaflet for specific disposal instructions. Some medications may have unique disposal requirements.

- Utilize local medication take-back programs or events, often organized by pharmacies or community health organizations, for safe disposal.

- If a take-back program is unavailable, follow the FDA guidelines for household disposal: mix medications (do not crush tablets or capsules) with an unpalatable substance like dirt, cat litter, or used coffee grounds.

- Place the mixture in a sealed plastic bag or container to prevent leakage and dispose of it in your household trash.

- Remove all personal information from medication bottles or packaging before disposal to protect your privacy.

- Avoid flushing medications down the toilet or sink unless specifically instructed by the medication label, as this can contaminate water supplies.

Common pitfalls

- Disposing of medications in the trash without mixing them with an unpalatable substance, increasing the risk of accidental ingestion by children or pets
- Forgetting to remove personal information from medication packaging, leading to potential privacy breaches

Progress tracking

- Monitor the frequency of medication disposal and ensure adherence to safe practices
- Evaluate the impact of proper disposal on household safety and environmental responsibility

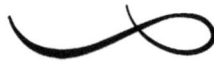

Chapter 18: Developing a Personal Action Plan

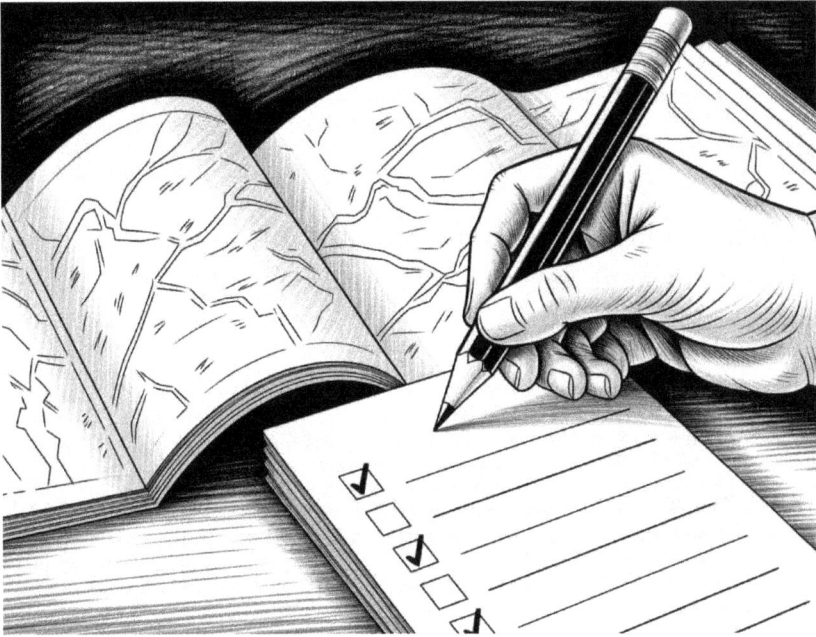

EXERCISE 79. PERSONAL HEALTH ASSESSMENT

Objective

Gain insight into your current health status to identify areas for improvement and set realistic goals for managing chronic diseases

Step-by-step instructions

- Gather recent medical records, including lab results, blood pressure readings, and any relevant imaging reports. Organize them in a folder or digital file for easy access.

- List all current medications, including dosages and frequency. Note any side effects or concerns you have experienced.

- Record your daily habits, such as diet, exercise, sleep patterns, and stress levels, for one week. Use a journal or app to track this information accurately.

- Identify any symptoms or health changes you have noticed recently. Be specific about their frequency, duration, and intensity.

- Evaluate your emotional well-being by noting feelings of anxiety, depression, or stress. Consider using a mood-tracking app or journal for detailed insights.

- Set up a meeting with your healthcare provider to review your findings. Prepare questions or topics you wish to discuss, focusing on areas where you seek improvement.

- Collaborate with your healthcare provider to develop a personalized action plan. Include specific, measurable goals and strategies for managing your chronic conditions effectively.

Common pitfalls

- Overlooking minor symptoms that may indicate changes in your health status
- Failing to track daily habits consistently, leading to incomplete data

Progress tracking

- Monitor changes in symptoms and overall health after implementing your action plan
- Regularly review and adjust your goals with your healthcare provider to ensure continued progress

EXERCISE 80. IDENTIFYING HEALTH PRIORITIES

Objective

Identify and prioritize key health areas to focus on for effective
management of chronic conditions

Step-by-step instructions

- List all chronic conditions you are currently managing,
  such as diabetes, hypertension, or musculoskeletal issues.
  Include any other health concerns that impact your daily
  life.

- Rank these conditions based on their impact on your
  quality of life. Consider factors like symptom severity,
  frequency, and how they affect your daily activities.

- Identify specific symptoms or challenges associated with
  each condition. Be detailed about how these symptoms
  manifest and their impact on your physical and
  emotional well-being.

- Reflect on your current management strategies for each
  condition. Note what is working well and where you face
  difficulties or need improvement.

- Set clear, achievable goals for each condition. Focus on
  areas where you can make the most significant impact on
  your health and quality of life.

- Prioritize these goals based on urgency and feasibility. Consider which goals will provide the most immediate benefits and which require longer-term commitment.

- Develop a plan to address your top priorities. Include specific actions, resources needed, and a timeline for implementation.

Common pitfalls

- Failing to consider the emotional impact of chronic conditions when prioritizing health areas
- Setting unrealistic goals that are difficult to achieve, leading to frustration and decreased motivation

Progress tracking

- Regularly review and adjust your priorities and goals as your health status and circumstances change
- Track improvements in symptoms and overall well-being to assess the effectiveness of your action plan

EXERCISE 81. SETTING REALISTIC HEALTH GOALS

Objective

Establish achievable health goals that align with your lifestyle and priorities to effectively manage chronic conditions

Step-by-step instructions

- Reflect on your current health status and identify areas where you want to see improvement. Consider aspects like blood sugar levels, blood pressure, physical activity, and pain management.

- Write down specific, measurable goals for each area. For example, aim to reduce your blood pressure by 10 mmHg or increase your daily steps by 2,000.

- Break down each goal into smaller, manageable steps. If your goal is to exercise more, start with a 10-minute walk three times a week and gradually increase the duration and frequency.

- Set a realistic timeline for achieving each goal. Consider your current commitments and choose a timeframe that allows for steady progress without overwhelming yourself.

- Identify potential obstacles that might hinder your progress, such as time constraints or lack of motivation. Develop strategies to overcome these challenges, like scheduling workouts in advance or finding a workout buddy.

- Track your progress regularly using a journal, app, or spreadsheet. Record your achievements and any setbacks to understand what works and what needs adjustment.

- Celebrate small victories along the way to maintain motivation. Reward yourself with non-food-related treats, like a new book or a relaxing activity, when you reach a milestone.

Common pitfalls

- Setting vague or overly ambitious goals that are difficult to measure or achieve
- Neglecting to adjust goals as your health status or circumstances change

Progress tracking

- Review your goals and progress monthly to ensure they remain relevant and achievable
- Adjust your action plan as needed to accommodate changes in your health or lifestyle

EXERCISE 82. CREATING A DAILY ROUTINE

Objective

Establish a consistent daily routine that supports effective self-management of chronic conditions

Step-by-step instructions

- Identify key activities that support your health, such as medication intake, meal planning, exercise, and relaxation techniques. List these activities in order of importance.

- Determine the best time of day for each activity based on your personal energy levels and daily schedule. For example, schedule exercise when you feel most energetic and plan meals around your work commitments.

- Allocate specific time slots for each activity, ensuring you have enough time to complete them without feeling rushed. Use a planner or digital calendar to block out these times.

- Incorporate flexibility into your routine to accommodate unexpected events or changes in your schedule. Have backup plans for essential activities, like a quick workout routine or a healthy meal option.

- Set reminders or alarms to prompt you to start each activity on time. Use smartphone apps or wearable devices to help you stay on track.

- Review your routine weekly to assess its effectiveness and make adjustments as needed. Consider factors like how well you adhered to the schedule and any challenges you faced.

- Gradually introduce new activities or habits that support your health goals, such as mindfulness practices or additional physical activity, as you become comfortable with your routine.

Common pitfalls

- Overloading your schedule with too many activities, leading to burnout
- Neglecting to adjust your routine as your health needs or lifestyle change

Progress tracking

- Keep a daily log of your activities and note any deviations from your routine
- Evaluate your adherence to the routine and its impact on your symptoms and overall well-being

EXERCISE 83. DEVELOPING A WEEKLY EXERCISE PLAN

Objective

Create a personalized weekly exercise plan that supports the management of diabetes, hypertension, and musculoskeletal issues

Step-by-step instructions

- Assess your current fitness level and any physical limitations. Consider factors like joint pain, fatigue, or cardiovascular concerns that may affect your ability to exercise.

- Consult with a healthcare professional to determine safe and effective exercise types for your condition. Options may include walking, swimming, cycling, or strength training.

- Set specific, realistic exercise goals for the week. Aim for at least 150 minutes of moderate-intensity aerobic activity, such as brisk walking, spread throughout the week.

- Choose a variety of exercises to target different muscle groups and prevent boredom. Include both aerobic activities and strength training exercises, like resistance bands or bodyweight exercises, twice a week.

- Schedule your workouts at times that fit your lifestyle and energy levels. Consider morning sessions if you feel more energetic or evening workouts if they help you unwind.

- Start each session with a 5-10 minute warm-up to prepare your body and reduce injury risk. Include light cardio and dynamic stretches.

- Gradually increase the intensity and duration of your workouts as your fitness improves. Add 5-10 minutes to your sessions every few weeks or increase resistance in strength exercises.

- Cool down after each workout with 5-10 minutes of stretching to enhance flexibility and aid recovery.

- Monitor your body's response to exercise, noting any pain or discomfort. Adjust your plan as needed to accommodate changes in your health or energy levels.

Common pitfalls

- Overexerting yourself by starting with high-intensity workouts
- Neglecting to incorporate rest days, leading to burnout or injury

Progress tracking

- Keep a weekly exercise log to track your activities, duration, and intensity
- Review your progress monthly to ensure your plan remains effective and aligned with your health goals

EXERCISE 84. PLANNING BALANCED MEALS

Objective

Create a balanced meal plan that supports the management of
diabetes, hypertension, and musculoskeletal issues

Step-by-step instructions

- Assess your dietary needs based on your chronic
  conditions. Consider factors like carbohydrate intake for
  diabetes, sodium levels for hypertension, and anti-
  inflammatory foods for musculoskeletal health.

- Consult with a healthcare professional or registered
  dietitian to determine appropriate portion sizes and food
  choices. Focus on whole grains, lean proteins, healthy
  fats, and a variety of fruits and vegetables.

- Plan your meals for the week, ensuring each meal
  includes a balance of macronutrients: carbohydrates,
  proteins, and fats. Aim for a plate that is half vegetables,
  a quarter protein, and a quarter whole grains.

- Incorporate foods rich in fiber, such as beans, lentils, and
  whole grains, to help manage blood sugar levels and
  support heart health.

- Limit processed foods and those high in added sugars
  and sodium. Opt for fresh or minimally processed
  options whenever possible.

- Prepare a shopping list based on your meal plan, focusing on seasonal and budget-friendly ingredients. Stick to the list to avoid impulse purchases.

- Allocate time for meal prep, such as chopping vegetables or cooking grains in advance, to streamline your cooking process during the week.

- Monitor your body's response to different foods, noting any changes in symptoms or energy levels. Adjust your meal plan as needed to better suit your health goals.

Common pitfalls

- Skipping meals or not eating at regular intervals, leading to blood sugar fluctuations
- Relying too heavily on convenience foods, which may be high in sodium and unhealthy fats

Progress tracking

- Keep a food diary to record your meals and any symptoms experienced
- Review your dietary habits monthly to ensure they align with your health objectives and make adjustments as necessary

EXERCISE 85. SCHEDULING REGULAR HEALTH CHECK-UPS

Objective

Create a personalized schedule for regular health check-ups to effectively manage diabetes, hypertension, and musculoskeletal issues

Step-by-step instructions

- Identify the specific health check-ups recommended for your conditions. Consult with your healthcare provider to determine necessary tests and frequency, such as blood glucose monitoring, blood pressure checks, and musculoskeletal assessments.

- Determine the optimal frequency for each type of check-up. For example, schedule blood glucose tests daily, blood pressure checks weekly, and musculoskeletal evaluations every six months.

- Choose convenient times for your appointments that align with your lifestyle and work schedule. Consider early morning or late afternoon slots to minimize disruption to your daily routine.

- Use a digital calendar or planner to set reminders for upcoming appointments. Include details like the type of check-up, location, and any preparation needed, such as fasting.

- Coordinate with your healthcare provider to ensure all necessary tests are scheduled in advance. Confirm appointments a week prior to avoid last-minute cancellations or rescheduling.

- Prepare a list of questions or concerns to discuss with your healthcare provider during each visit. Focus on changes in symptoms, medication side effects, or lifestyle adjustments.

- Keep a record of your test results and any recommendations from your healthcare provider. Use this information to track your progress and make informed decisions about your health management plan.

Common pitfalls

- Forgetting to schedule follow-up appointments, leading to gaps in monitoring
- Overlooking the importance of regular check-ups due to a busy lifestyle

Progress tracking

- Maintain a log of completed check-ups and upcoming appointments
- Review your health records quarterly to ensure all necessary tests are up-to-date and adjust your schedule as needed

EXERCISE 86. STRESS MANAGEMENT TECHNIQUES

Objective

Implement stress management techniques to improve overall well-being and support chronic disease management

Step-by-step instructions

- Identify stressors in your daily life by keeping a journal for one week. Note situations, people, or tasks that trigger stress responses.

- Choose a stress management technique that resonates with you, such as deep breathing, meditation, or progressive muscle relaxation. Allocate 10-15 minutes daily to practice this technique.

- Create a calming environment for your practice. Find a quiet space, dim the lights, and eliminate distractions like phones or loud noises.

- Incorporate physical activity into your routine, such as a 30-minute walk or yoga session, at least three times a week to help reduce stress levels.

- Establish a regular sleep schedule by going to bed and waking up at the same time each day. Aim for 7-9 hours of quality sleep to support stress reduction.

- Practice mindfulness by focusing on the present moment during daily activities. Use techniques like mindful eating or mindful breathing to enhance awareness and reduce stress.

- Connect with supportive friends or family members regularly. Share your experiences and seek encouragement to help manage stress effectively.

Common pitfalls

- Neglecting to prioritize stress management due to a busy schedule
- Relying solely on one technique without exploring other options that may be more effective

Progress tracking

- Maintain a stress journal to record your stress levels and the effectiveness of different techniques
- Review your journal monthly to identify patterns and adjust your stress management plan as needed

EXERCISE 87. BUILDING A SUPPORT SYSTEM

Objective

Establish a reliable support system to enhance self-management of chronic diseases

Step-by-step instructions

- Identify key individuals in your life who can provide support, such as family members, friends, or colleagues. Consider those who are understanding, reliable, and willing to assist you in managing your condition.

- Communicate your needs clearly to your support network. Explain your chronic condition, the challenges you face, and how they can help, whether it's through emotional support, practical assistance, or accountability.

- Schedule regular check-ins with your support system. Set up weekly or bi-weekly meetings, either in person or virtually, to discuss your progress, challenges, and any adjustments needed in your management plan.

- Join a local or online support group for individuals with similar chronic conditions. Participate in discussions, share experiences, and learn from others who are managing diabetes, hypertension, or musculoskeletal issues.

- Utilize technology to stay connected with your support network. Use messaging apps, video calls, or social media to maintain regular communication and share updates on your health journey.

- Encourage your support system to educate themselves about your condition. Provide them with resources, such as articles or books, to help them understand your needs better and offer more informed support.

- Express gratitude to your support network regularly. Acknowledge their efforts and let them know how much their support means to you, fostering a positive and encouraging environment.

Common pitfalls

- Relying solely on one person for support, which can lead to burnout or strained relationships
- Failing to communicate changes in your condition or needs to your support network

Progress tracking

- Keep a journal of interactions with your support system, noting helpful advice or actions
- Review your support system's effectiveness quarterly and make adjustments as needed to ensure continued benefit

EXERCISE 88. MONITORING HEALTH PROGRESS

Objective

Track and evaluate your health progress to enhance self-management of chronic diseases

Step-by-step instructions

- Set specific, measurable health goals related to your chronic condition, such as maintaining a target blood sugar level, reducing blood pressure, or improving joint flexibility.

- Choose appropriate tools for monitoring your health, such as a blood glucose meter, blood pressure monitor, or a fitness tracker. Ensure these tools are calibrated and used correctly.

- Record your health data consistently. For diabetes, log blood sugar levels daily. For hypertension, measure blood pressure at least twice a week. For musculoskeletal issues, track pain levels and mobility daily.

- Review your recorded data weekly to identify trends or patterns. Look for improvements, setbacks, or any irregularities that may require attention.

- Adjust your management plan based on your findings. If blood sugar levels are consistently high, consider dietary changes. If blood pressure is elevated, evaluate stress management techniques or medication adherence.

- Schedule regular appointments with healthcare professionals to discuss your progress and any necessary adjustments to your treatment plan.

- Celebrate small victories and improvements to maintain motivation and a positive mindset.

Common pitfalls

- Inconsistent data recording, leading to inaccurate assessments
- Ignoring small changes in health metrics that could indicate larger issues

Progress tracking

- Maintain a health journal or digital app to log daily measurements and observations
- Review your progress monthly with a healthcare professional to ensure your management plan remains effective

EXERCISE 89. ADJUSTING HEALTH STRATEGIES

Objective

Adapt your health management strategies to better fit your lifestyle and improve chronic disease control

Step-by-step instructions

- Assess your current health management plan. Identify which strategies are working well and which are not yielding desired results.

- Reflect on recent lifestyle changes, such as work schedule adjustments, family commitments, or new stressors, that may impact your health management.

- Prioritize areas needing improvement. Focus on one or two key aspects, such as diet, exercise, or medication adherence, that require immediate attention.

- Research alternative strategies or tools that align with your current lifestyle. Consider options like meal delivery services, home workout apps, or medication reminders.

- Consult with healthcare professionals to discuss potential adjustments. Seek their advice on safe and effective modifications to your management plan.

- Implement changes gradually. Introduce one new strategy at a time to avoid overwhelming yourself and to accurately assess its effectiveness.

- Monitor the impact of each change on your health metrics. Use tools like a health journal or digital app to track progress and make data-driven decisions.

- Re-evaluate your plan monthly. Adjust strategies as needed to ensure they continue to support your health goals and fit your lifestyle.

Common pitfalls

- Making too many changes at once, leading to confusion and difficulty in tracking effectiveness
- Neglecting to consult healthcare professionals before making significant adjustments

Progress tracking

- Use a checklist to track the implementation of new strategies and their outcomes
- Schedule monthly reviews with a healthcare professional to discuss progress and refine your plan

EXERCISE 90. CELEBRATING HEALTH ACHIEVEMENTS

Objective

Recognize and celebrate personal health achievements to foster a positive mindset and enhance motivation for managing chronic diseases

Step-by-step instructions

- Identify specific health milestones you have achieved, such as reaching a target blood sugar level, lowering blood pressure, or increasing physical activity.

- Reflect on the efforts and strategies that led to these achievements. Consider lifestyle changes, dietary adjustments, or exercise routines that contributed to your success.

- Choose a meaningful way to celebrate your accomplishments. Options could include treating yourself to a favorite activity, sharing your success with friends or family, or rewarding yourself with a small gift.

- Document your achievements in a health journal or digital app. Include details about the milestone, how you achieved it, and how you celebrated.

- Share your success with your healthcare team during your next appointment. Discuss the positive impact of your achievements on your overall health management plan.

- Set new health goals to continue your progress. Use your past achievements as motivation to tackle new challenges and maintain a positive outlook.

- Regularly review and update your list of achievements. Reflect on your journey and use it as a source of inspiration during challenging times.

Common pitfalls

- Failing to acknowledge small achievements, which can lead to decreased motivation
- Comparing your progress to others, rather than focusing on personal growth

Progress tracking

- Maintain a dedicated section in your health journal for recording achievements and celebrations
- Review your list of achievements monthly to reinforce a positive mindset and motivate continued progress

EXERCISE 91. REFLECTING ON HEALTH JOURNEY

Objective

Gain insight into your health journey to enhance self-awareness and empower effective self-management

Step-by-step instructions

- Set aside 15-30 minutes in a quiet space to reflect on your health journey. Ensure you have a notebook or digital device for recording your thoughts.

- Begin by recalling the initial diagnosis of your chronic condition. Note your feelings, concerns, and any immediate actions you took.

- Identify key moments or turning points in your health journey. Consider changes in symptoms, lifestyle adjustments, or significant medical appointments.

- Reflect on the strategies and tools you have used to manage your condition. Evaluate their effectiveness and note any adjustments you made over time.

- Consider the support systems that have been beneficial, such as family, friends, or healthcare professionals. Reflect on how they have contributed to your journey.

- Acknowledge challenges you have faced and how you overcame them. Identify any patterns or recurring obstacles that may need further attention.

- Write down lessons learned from your experiences. Focus on insights that have positively influenced your self-management and overall well-being.

- Conclude by setting a personal intention or goal for the next phase of your health journey. Ensure it is specific, measurable, and aligned with your current needs.

Common pitfalls

- Focusing solely on negative experiences, which can hinder motivation and progress
- Overlooking small victories and incremental improvements

Progress tracking

- Maintain a dedicated section in your health journal for ongoing reflections and insights
- Review your reflections quarterly to identify patterns and adjust your management strategies accordingly

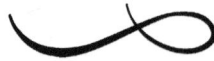

Chapter 19: Staying Motivated for Long-Term Exercise

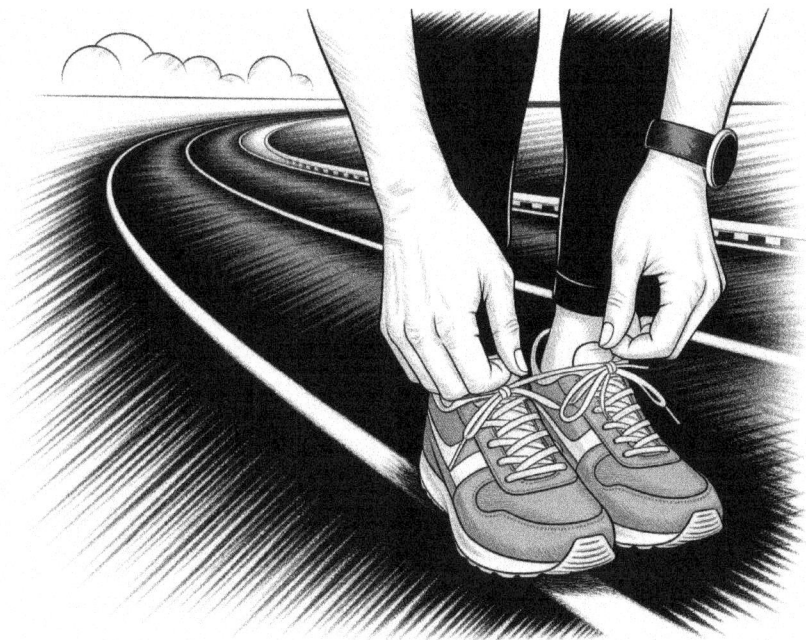

EXERCISE 92. SETTING LONG-TERM HEALTH GOALS

Objective

Establish and maintain long-term health goals to enhance self-management and improve quality of life

Step-by-step instructions

- Reflect on your current health status and identify areas for improvement. Consider factors such as blood sugar levels, blood pressure, physical activity, and pain management.

- Set specific, measurable, achievable, relevant, and time-bound (SMART) goals. For example, aim to walk 30 minutes a day, five times a week, or reduce sodium intake by 20% over the next month.

- Break down each goal into smaller, manageable steps. If your goal is to increase physical activity, start with a 10-minute walk three times a week and gradually increase the duration and frequency.

- Identify potential obstacles and plan strategies to overcome them. Consider time constraints, financial limitations, or lack of motivation, and develop solutions such as scheduling workouts or finding cost-effective meal plans.

- Create a visual representation of your goals, such as a chart or vision board, to keep them top of mind. Place it in a prominent location as a daily reminder of your commitment.

- Regularly review and adjust your goals based on progress and changing circumstances. Be flexible and willing to modify your approach if necessary to stay on track.

- Celebrate milestones and achievements along the way. Recognize your efforts and reward yourself with non-food-related treats, such as a new book or a relaxing day out.

Common pitfalls

- Setting unrealistic goals that lead to frustration and discouragement
- Neglecting to adjust goals as circumstances change, resulting in stagnation

Progress tracking

- Use a health journal or digital app to record your goals, progress, and any adjustments made
- Review your progress monthly to ensure alignment with your long-term health objectives

EXERCISE 93. CREATING A VISION BOARD

Objective

Cultivate a positive mindset and reinforce motivation for managing chronic diseases through visual inspiration

Step-by-step instructions

- Gather materials such as magazines, scissors, glue, and a large poster board or corkboard. Alternatively, use a digital platform or app for creating vision boards.

- Set aside 30-60 minutes in a quiet, comfortable space to focus on your vision board. Ensure you have access to your materials or digital tools.

- Reflect on your health goals and aspirations. Consider aspects such as improved energy levels, better symptom management, or enhanced physical activity.

- Search for images, words, or phrases that resonate with your health objectives. Look for visuals that evoke positive emotions and align with your desired outcomes.

- Arrange the selected images and words on your board in a way that feels meaningful and inspiring. Consider grouping similar themes together for clarity.

- Secure the images and words to your board using glue or pins. If using a digital platform, organize the elements in a visually appealing layout.

- Place your completed vision board in a prominent location where you will see it daily, such as your bedroom, office, or kitchen.

- Spend a few moments each day reflecting on your vision board. Allow it to remind you of your goals and motivate you to take consistent action.

Common pitfalls

- Overloading the board with too many elements, which can dilute focus and clarity
- Choosing images or words that do not genuinely resonate with personal goals

Progress tracking

- Take a photo of your vision board for reference and comparison over time
- Review and update your board every 3-6 months to reflect evolving goals and achievements

EXERCISE 94. DEVELOPING A REWARD SYSTEM

Objective

Create a personalized reward system to maintain motivation
and reinforce positive behaviors in managing chronic diseases

Step-by-step instructions

- Identify specific behaviors or milestones you want to
  reward. Consider actions like consistently monitoring
  blood sugar, maintaining a low-sodium diet, or
  completing a weekly exercise routine.

- Choose rewards that are meaningful and motivating to
  you. Opt for non-food-related rewards such as a new
  book, a movie night, or a relaxing bath.

- Set clear criteria for earning each reward. For example,
  reward yourself with a new book after two weeks of daily
  blood pressure monitoring or a movie night after
  completing a month of regular exercise.

- Create a visual chart or list to track your progress and
  rewards. Display it in a visible location to remind you of
  your goals and incentives.

- Share your reward system with a friend or family
  member for accountability. They can help celebrate your
  achievements and encourage you to stay on track.

- Regularly review and adjust your reward system to
  ensure it remains motivating. As you achieve goals, set

new ones and update rewards to match your evolving interests and needs.

Common pitfalls

- Choosing rewards that conflict with health goals, such as unhealthy food treats
- Setting rewards that are too difficult to achieve, leading to frustration

Progress tracking

- Use a journal or app to log completed tasks and earned rewards
- Review your reward system monthly to ensure it aligns with your current health objectives and motivation levels

EXERCISE 95. TRACKING PROGRESS WITH A JOURNAL

Objective

Enhance self-awareness and track progress in managing chronic diseases through consistent journaling

Step-by-step instructions

- Choose a journal format that suits your lifestyle, such as a physical notebook, a digital app, or a spreadsheet.

- Set aside 5-10 minutes daily to write in your journal. Select a consistent time, like after breakfast or before bed, to establish a routine.

- Record key health metrics relevant to your condition, such as blood sugar levels, blood pressure readings, or pain levels.

- Note any lifestyle factors that may influence your health, including diet, physical activity, stress levels, and sleep quality.

- Reflect on your emotional state and any challenges or successes you experienced that day in managing your condition.

- Set small, achievable goals for the next day or week, focusing on areas where you want to improve or maintain progress.

- Review your entries weekly to identify patterns, triggers, or areas for improvement. Use this insight to adjust your management strategies.

Common pitfalls

- Inconsistent journaling, which can lead to incomplete data and missed insights
- Focusing only on negative aspects, which can undermine motivation

Progress tracking

- Use your journal to compare current entries with past ones, noting improvements or setbacks
- Share your journal insights with healthcare professionals to enhance your treatment plan

EXERCISE 96. FINDING AN ACCOUNTABILITY PARTNER

Objective

Establish a supportive relationship to enhance motivation and accountability in managing chronic diseases

Step-by-step instructions

- Identify potential accountability partners among friends, family, or support groups. Consider individuals who understand your health goals and can provide encouragement.

- Discuss your health objectives and management strategies with your chosen partner. Ensure they are comfortable with the level of involvement you expect.

- Set clear expectations for communication frequency and methods. Decide whether you will check in daily, weekly, or at other intervals, and whether you will use phone calls, texts, or in-person meetings.

- Share specific goals and progress updates with your partner. Be open about challenges and successes to foster a transparent and supportive relationship.

- Encourage your partner to share their own health goals, if applicable. This mutual exchange can strengthen the partnership and provide additional motivation.

- Regularly review the effectiveness of the partnership. Adjust communication methods or frequency as needed to maintain motivation and support.

Common pitfalls

- Choosing a partner who is not fully committed or lacks understanding of your health challenges
- Failing to communicate openly, leading to misunderstandings or reduced support

Progress tracking

- Keep a log of check-ins and discussions with your accountability partner
- Reflect on how the partnership impacts your motivation and progress in managing your condition

EXERCISE 97. JOINING A SUPPORT GROUP

Objective

Enhance emotional support and gain practical insights for managing chronic diseases through participation in a support group

Step-by-step instructions

- Research local or online support groups focused on diabetes, hypertension, or musculoskeletal issues. Use resources like community centers, hospitals, or online platforms.

- Evaluate the group's format and schedule to ensure it fits your lifestyle. Consider whether you prefer in-person meetings, virtual sessions, or a combination of both.

- Attend an initial meeting to assess the group's dynamics and determine if it aligns with your needs and values. Observe the level of engagement and support among members.

- Actively participate by sharing your experiences and challenges. Be open to receiving advice and learning from others' experiences.

- Establish connections with group members who share similar goals or challenges. Exchange contact information to foster relationships outside of meetings.

- Regularly attend meetings to maintain a sense of community and accountability. Consistency can enhance the benefits of group support.

- Reflect on the insights and strategies gained from the group. Implement applicable advice into your daily management routine.

Common pitfalls

- Joining a group that lacks structure or focus, which can lead to unproductive sessions
- Being hesitant to share personal experiences, limiting the potential for support and learning

Progress tracking

- Keep a record of the strategies and advice gained from the group
- Monitor changes in your condition and emotional well-being as a result of group participation

EXERCISE 98. EXPLORING NEW PHYSICAL ACTIVITIES

Objective

Discover and incorporate new physical activities to enhance motivation and support chronic disease management

Step-by-step instructions

- Assess your current physical activity level and identify any limitations related to your chronic condition. Consider factors such as time availability, physical ability, and personal interests.

- Research various physical activities that are suitable for individuals with diabetes, hypertension, or musculoskeletal issues. Look for activities that are low-impact, enjoyable, and can be easily integrated into your routine.

- Choose one or two new activities to try. Examples include yoga, swimming, cycling, or walking. Ensure the activities align with your health goals and physical capabilities.

- Set a realistic schedule for incorporating the new activities into your weekly routine. Aim for at least 150 minutes of moderate-intensity exercise per week, as recommended by health guidelines.

- Start slowly and gradually increase the duration and intensity of the activities as your comfort and fitness level improve. Listen to your body and adjust as needed to prevent injury.

- Track your progress by keeping a log of the activities you engage in, noting the duration, intensity, and any physical or emotional changes you experience.

- Reflect on how the new activities impact your overall well-being and chronic disease management. Adjust your routine as necessary to maintain motivation and effectiveness.

Common pitfalls

- Choosing activities that are too intense or unsuitable for your condition, leading to discomfort or injury
- Failing to schedule regular time for new activities, resulting in inconsistent participation

Progress tracking

- Maintain a journal of your physical activity, noting improvements in energy levels, mood, and symptom management
- Regularly review your activity log to identify patterns and make informed adjustments to your routine

EXERCISE 99. SCHEDULING REGULAR CHECK-INS

Objective

Establish a routine for regular self-assessment and communication with healthcare providers to enhance chronic disease management

Step-by-step instructions

- Identify the key aspects of your condition that require regular monitoring, such as blood sugar levels, blood pressure, or joint pain.

- Determine the frequency of check-ins needed for each aspect, based on your healthcare provider's recommendations. This could be daily, weekly, or monthly.

- Use a calendar or digital planner to schedule these check-ins. Set reminders to ensure consistency and prevent missed assessments.

- Prepare a checklist of questions or topics to discuss during each check-in. Include any changes in symptoms, medication side effects, or lifestyle adjustments.

- Allocate time for self-reflection before each check-in. Consider how your condition has impacted your daily life and any challenges you've faced.

- Document the outcomes of each check-in, noting any changes in your condition or treatment plan. Use a journal or digital app for easy tracking.

- Share your findings with your healthcare provider during appointments. Use this information to collaboratively adjust your management plan as needed.

Common pitfalls

- Neglecting to schedule check-ins, leading to inconsistent monitoring and management
- Failing to prepare adequately for check-ins, resulting in incomplete assessments

Progress tracking

- Maintain a log of check-in outcomes and any adjustments made to your management plan
- Review your log regularly to identify patterns and areas for improvement

EXERCISE 100. PRACTICING POSITIVE SELF-TALK

Objective

Cultivate a habit of positive self-talk to enhance self-management and motivation in managing chronic diseases

Step-by-step instructions

- Identify negative self-talk patterns by paying attention to your thoughts throughout the day. Note any recurring negative phrases or beliefs related to your health condition.

- Challenge these negative thoughts by questioning their validity. Ask yourself if they are based on facts or assumptions, and consider alternative, more positive perspectives.

- Create a list of positive affirmations that counteract the negative thoughts. Ensure these affirmations are realistic, specific, and focused on your strengths and capabilities.

- Set aside a few minutes each day to practice these affirmations. Repeat them aloud or write them down, ideally in the morning or before bed, to reinforce a positive mindset.

- Incorporate positive self-talk into your daily routine by using affirmations during challenging moments, such as before a medical appointment or when experiencing symptoms.

- Reflect on the impact of positive self-talk by keeping a journal of your experiences. Note any changes in your mood, motivation, or symptom management.

- Adjust your affirmations as needed to address new challenges or goals, ensuring they remain relevant and supportive of your self-management efforts.

Common pitfalls

- Using affirmations that are too vague or unrealistic, leading to frustration or disbelief
- Neglecting to practice positive self-talk consistently, resulting in limited impact

Progress tracking

- Maintain a journal of your affirmations and any changes in your mindset or condition
- Regularly review your journal to identify patterns and make informed adjustments to your affirmations

EXERCISE 101. VISUALIZING SUCCESS

Objective

Develop a clear vision of success to enhance motivation and self-management in managing chronic diseases

Step-by-step instructions

- Find a quiet space where you can relax without distractions. Sit comfortably and close your eyes.

- Take a few deep breaths to center yourself. Focus on your breathing to calm your mind.

- Visualize a day in your life where you are successfully managing your chronic condition. Imagine waking up feeling energized and ready to take on the day.

- Picture yourself engaging in healthy habits, such as preparing a nutritious meal, exercising, or monitoring your health metrics. See yourself doing these activities with ease and confidence.

- Envision the positive outcomes of your efforts, such as improved energy levels, reduced symptoms, or a sense of accomplishment. Focus on the emotions you feel in this successful scenario.

- Create a mental image of yourself interacting with healthcare providers, feeling empowered and informed. Imagine discussing your progress and collaboratively planning your next steps.

- Spend a few minutes each day revisiting this visualization. Use it as a motivational tool to reinforce your commitment to self-management and to remind yourself of the benefits of your efforts.

Common pitfalls

- Allowing negative thoughts to interrupt your visualization, diminishing its effectiveness
- Skipping daily practice, leading to reduced impact on motivation and mindset

Progress tracking

- Keep a journal of your visualization experiences and any changes in your motivation or condition
- Regularly review your journal to identify patterns and make informed adjustments to your visualization practice

EXERCISE 102. OVERCOMING SETBACKS

Objective

Develop resilience and adaptability to effectively manage setbacks in chronic disease management

Step-by-step instructions

- Acknowledge the setback by identifying what went wrong and how it impacted your health management. Be specific about the situation and your feelings.

- Reframe the setback as a learning opportunity. Consider what you can learn from the experience and how it can inform your future actions.

- Set a small, achievable goal to regain momentum. Focus on a specific aspect of your health management, such as taking a short walk or preparing a healthy meal.

- Create a plan to address the setback. Outline the steps you will take to overcome the challenge and prevent similar issues in the future.

- Seek support from friends, family, or healthcare professionals. Share your experience and ask for advice or encouragement to help you stay motivated.

- Practice self-compassion by reminding yourself that setbacks are a normal part of the journey. Avoid self-criticism and focus on your progress and strengths.

- Reflect on your progress by keeping a journal of your experiences. Note any improvements in your mindset, motivation, or symptom management.

Common pitfalls

- Dwelling on the setback without taking action to move forward
- Setting unrealistic goals that lead to further frustration

Progress tracking

- Maintain a journal of setbacks and your responses to them
- Regularly review your journal to identify patterns and make informed adjustments to your strategies

EXERCISE 103. CELEBRATING SMALL WINS

Objective

Recognize and celebrate small achievements to boost motivation
and maintain a positive mindset in managing chronic diseases

Step-by-step instructions

- Identify a small goal related to your health management,
  such as drinking an extra glass of water daily or taking a
  10-minute walk.

- Track your progress by noting each time you achieve this
  goal. Use a journal, app, or calendar to record your
  successes.

- Choose a simple reward for reaching your goal
  consistently, like enjoying a favorite hobby or spending
  time with a loved one.

- Share your achievement with a friend, family member, or
  support group to reinforce your success and gain
  encouragement.

- Reflect on how achieving this small goal contributes to
  your overall health management and well-being.

- Set a new small goal once the current one becomes a
  habit, gradually building on your successes.

Common pitfalls

- Overlooking small achievements and focusing only on larger goals
- Setting goals that are too ambitious, leading to frustration

Progress tracking

- Maintain a log of your small goals and achievements
- Regularly review your log to recognize patterns and adjust your goals accordingly

EXERCISE 104. REFLECTING ON PERSONAL GROWTH

Objective

Cultivate a mindset of continuous personal growth to enhance self-management of chronic diseases

Step-by-step instructions

- Set aside 10 minutes each day for reflection. Find a quiet space where you can focus without distractions.

- Think about a recent experience related to managing your condition. Consider what went well and what could be improved.

- Identify one area where you have made progress, no matter how small. Acknowledge this achievement and how it contributes to your overall health journey.

- Consider a challenge you faced and how you responded. Reflect on what you learned from this experience and how it can guide future actions.

- Write down your reflections in a journal. Include both positive developments and areas for improvement to track your growth over time.

- Set a small, specific goal for the coming week based on your reflections. Ensure it is achievable and directly related to managing your condition.

- Review your journal entries weekly to recognize patterns and adjust your strategies as needed.

Common pitfalls

- Focusing only on negative experiences without acknowledging progress
- Setting goals that are too broad or unrealistic

Progress tracking

- Maintain a journal of daily reflections and weekly goals
- Regularly review your journal to identify growth and areas for further development

EXERCISE 105. REASSESSING MOTIVATION FACTORS

Objective

Identify and reassess personal motivation factors to sustain long-term self-management of chronic diseases

Step-by-step instructions

- Set aside 15 minutes in a quiet space to reflect on your current motivations for managing your health.

- List three primary reasons why managing your condition is important to you. Consider aspects like family, career, or personal well-being.

- Evaluate each reason by asking yourself how it impacts your daily life and long-term goals. Consider both emotional and practical aspects.

- Rank these motivations in order of importance to you. Reflect on why the top reason holds the most significance.

- Identify any changes in your life that might have shifted your motivations. Consider new responsibilities, relationships, or health developments.

- Adjust your health management strategies to align with your current motivations. Ensure they are realistic and achievable within your lifestyle.

- Revisit this exercise monthly to ensure your motivations remain relevant and continue to drive your self-management efforts.

Common pitfalls

- Failing to recognize changes in personal motivations over time
- Ignoring emotional factors that influence motivation

Progress tracking

- Maintain a journal of your motivations and any changes over time
- Regularly review and update your motivations to stay aligned with your health goals

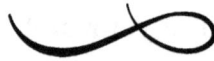

Chapter 20: Coping with Setbacks Exercise

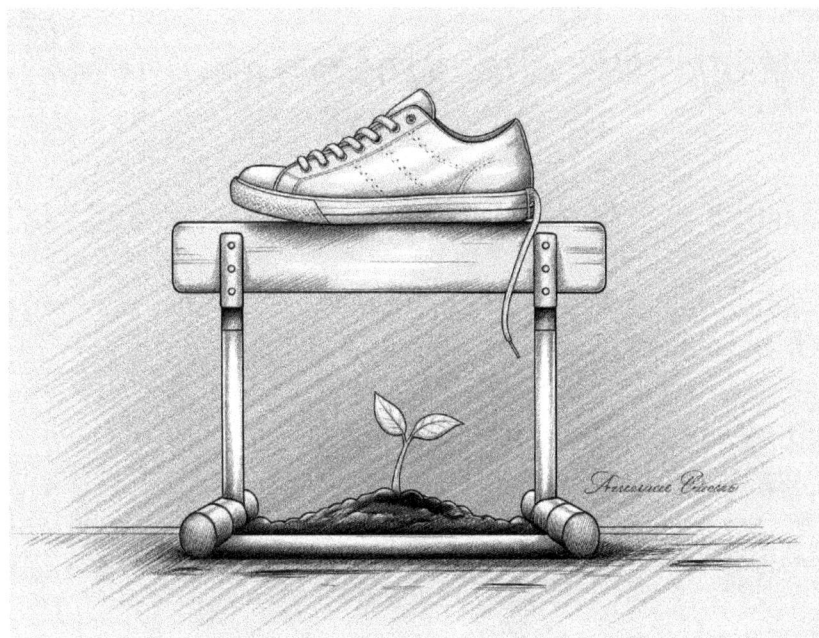

EXERCISE 106. IDENTIFYING EMOTIONAL TRIGGERS

Objective

Recognize and understand emotional triggers that may impact the management of chronic diseases

Step-by-step instructions

- Set aside 20 minutes in a quiet, comfortable space where you can focus without interruptions.

- Reflect on recent situations where you felt a strong emotional response related to managing your condition. Consider both positive and negative emotions.

- Write down three specific instances where your emotions influenced your health management decisions. Include details about the situation, your emotional response, and the outcome.

- Identify common themes or patterns in these instances. Look for triggers such as stress, fatigue, or specific interactions with others.

- Rank these emotional triggers in order of how frequently they occur or how strongly they impact your health management.

- Develop a plan to address each trigger. Consider strategies like deep breathing, taking a short walk, or reaching out to a supportive friend.

- Practice these strategies the next time you encounter an emotional trigger. Observe how they affect your response and adjust as needed.

Common pitfalls

- Ignoring subtle emotional responses that may still impact decision-making
- Focusing only on negative emotions without recognizing positive influences

Progress tracking

- Maintain a journal of emotional triggers and your responses
- Regularly review your journal to identify improvements and areas needing further attention

EXERCISE 107. PRACTICING SELF-COMPASSION

Objective

Cultivate self-compassion to enhance resilience and improve self-management of chronic diseases

Step-by-step instructions

- Set aside 10 minutes in a quiet, comfortable space where you can focus without distractions.

- Reflect on a recent situation where you felt you fell short in managing your condition. Consider the emotions and thoughts that arose.

- Write down a brief description of the situation, including what happened and how you felt.

- Imagine a close friend is in the same situation. Write a compassionate response you would offer them, focusing on understanding and support.

- Read your compassionate response aloud to yourself, applying the same kindness to your own experience.

- Identify one positive action you can take to address the situation or prevent it in the future. Write it down and commit to implementing it.

- Practice this exercise weekly to build a habit of self-compassion and reinforce positive self-management behaviors.

Common pitfalls

- Being overly critical of oneself instead of focusing on understanding and growth
- Neglecting to follow through with the positive action identified

Progress tracking

- Maintain a journal of situations and your compassionate responses
- Review your journal monthly to observe patterns and improvements in self-compassion

EXERCISE 108. DEVELOPING A POSITIVE MINDSET

Objective

Foster a positive mindset to enhance self-management of chronic diseases

Step-by-step instructions

- Dedicate 15 minutes each morning to a quiet space where you can focus on your thoughts.

- Begin by taking five deep breaths, inhaling through your nose and exhaling through your mouth, to center yourself.

- Reflect on three things you are grateful for in your life, related or unrelated to your health. Write them down in a journal.

- Identify one positive affirmation that resonates with you, such as "I am capable of managing my health effectively." Repeat it aloud five times.

- Visualize a successful day of managing your condition, including specific actions you will take to maintain your health.

- Set one achievable goal for the day that supports your health management, such as preparing a healthy meal or taking a 20-minute walk.

- At the end of the day, review your goal and note any progress or challenges in your journal.

Common pitfalls

- Skipping the exercise due to a busy schedule
- Focusing on negative thoughts instead of positive affirmations

Progress tracking

- Maintain a daily journal of your gratitude reflections, affirmations, and goals
- Review your journal weekly to identify patterns and areas for improvement

EXERCISE 109. BUILDING RESILIENCE

Objective

Enhance resilience to effectively manage chronic diseases and navigate daily challenges

Step-by-step instructions

- Allocate 15 minutes in a quiet, comfortable space where you can focus without interruptions.

- Begin by taking five deep breaths, inhaling through your nose and exhaling through your mouth, to center yourself.

- Reflect on a recent challenge you faced in managing your condition. Consider the emotions and thoughts that arose.

- Write down a brief description of the challenge, including what happened and how you felt.

- Identify one lesson or positive aspect you can extract from the experience, such as increased awareness or a new strategy.

- Visualize yourself successfully overcoming a similar challenge in the future, using the lesson or positive aspect identified.

- Commit to one action that will help you apply this lesson in your daily management routine. Write it down and plan to implement it.

- Practice this exercise weekly to build resilience and reinforce effective self-management behaviors

Common pitfalls

- Focusing solely on negative aspects of the challenge instead of identifying positive lessons
- Neglecting to implement the action identified for future improvement

Progress tracking

- Maintain a journal of challenges, lessons learned, and actions taken
- Review your journal monthly to observe patterns and improvements in resilience

EXERCISE 110. STRESS REDUCTION TECHNIQUES

Objective

Reduce stress to improve self-management of chronic diseases

Step-by-step instructions

- Find a quiet, comfortable space where you can relax without interruptions for 10 minutes.

- Begin by taking five deep breaths, inhaling through your nose and exhaling through your mouth, to calm your mind.

- Close your eyes and focus on relaxing each part of your body, starting from your toes and moving up to your head. Spend about 30 seconds on each area.

- Visualize a peaceful scene, such as a beach or a forest, and imagine yourself there, feeling calm and at ease.

- Practice progressive muscle relaxation by tensing each muscle group for five seconds, then releasing. Start with your feet and work your way up to your shoulders.

- End the session by taking five more deep breaths, slowly opening your eyes, and returning to your day with a sense of calm.

Common pitfalls

- Allowing distractions to interrupt the relaxation process
- Rushing through the exercise without fully engaging in each step

Progress tracking

- Keep a journal of your stress levels before and after each session
- Review your journal weekly to identify improvements in stress management and overall well-being

EXERCISE 111. MINDFUL BREATHING EXERCISES

Objective

Enhance focus and reduce stress to support effective self-management of chronic diseases

Step-by-step instructions

- Find a quiet, comfortable space where you can sit or lie down without interruptions for 10 minutes.

- Close your eyes and take a deep breath in through your nose, allowing your abdomen to expand. Hold for a moment.

- Exhale slowly through your mouth, letting go of any tension. Repeat this deep breathing cycle five times.

- Shift your focus to your natural breathing rhythm. Notice the sensation of air entering and leaving your nostrils.

- If your mind starts to wander, gently bring your attention back to your breath without judgment.

- Continue this mindful breathing for 5-10 minutes, maintaining a relaxed and focused state.

- Gradually bring your awareness back to the present moment by wiggling your fingers and toes, then slowly open your eyes.

Common pitfalls

- Allowing distractions to break your focus
- Becoming frustrated with wandering thoughts instead of gently refocusing

Progress tracking

- Keep a journal of your stress levels before and after each session
- Review your journal weekly to identify improvements in focus and stress management

EXERCISE 112. JOURNALING FOR EMOTIONAL CLARITY

Objective

Gain emotional clarity to support effective self-management of chronic diseases

Step-by-step instructions

- Set aside 10-15 minutes each day for journaling in a quiet, comfortable space.

- Begin by writing down any emotions or thoughts that are currently on your mind. Be honest and open with yourself.

- Reflect on any recent events or interactions that may have triggered these emotions. Write about how they made you feel and why.

- Consider how these emotions might be affecting your management of your chronic condition. Note any patterns or recurring themes.

- Write about any positive experiences or achievements from the day, no matter how small. Focus on gratitude and personal growth.

- End your journaling session by setting a small, achievable goal for the next day related to your self-management.

Common pitfalls

- Skipping journaling sessions due to a busy schedule
- Focusing only on negative emotions without acknowledging positive experiences

Progress tracking

- Review your journal entries weekly to identify emotional patterns and their impact on your condition management
- Note any improvements in emotional clarity and self-management over time

EXERCISE 113. SETTING REALISTIC EXPECTATIONS

Objective

Develop a balanced perspective to enhance self-management of chronic diseases

Step-by-step instructions

- Set aside 15 minutes in a quiet space with a notebook or digital device.

- Write down your current expectations regarding the management of your chronic condition. Be specific about what you hope to achieve in the short and long term.

- Reflect on past experiences where you set expectations. Note any instances where expectations were met, exceeded, or fell short.

- Identify any unrealistic expectations by considering factors such as time, resources, and personal limitations. Adjust these expectations to be more achievable.

- Break down your adjusted expectations into smaller, manageable goals. Ensure each goal is specific, measurable, and time-bound.

- Prioritize these goals based on their impact on your health and quality of life. Focus on one or two goals at a time to avoid feeling overwhelmed.

- Revisit and revise your expectations regularly, especially after significant changes in your condition or lifestyle.

Common pitfalls

- Setting overly ambitious goals without considering personal limitations
- Neglecting to adjust expectations after changes in health status

Progress tracking

- Keep a record of your expectations and goals, noting any adjustments made over time
- Review your progress monthly to assess the realism of your expectations and make necessary changes

EXERCISE 114. CREATING A SUPPORTIVE ENVIRONMENT

Objective

Foster a supportive environment to enhance self-management of chronic diseases

Step-by-step instructions

- Identify key areas in your home where you spend the most time. Consider spaces like the kitchen, living room, and bedroom.

- Evaluate these areas for any potential stressors or obstacles that may hinder your self-management efforts. Look for clutter, lack of organization, or distractions.

- Make a list of changes that could create a more supportive environment. This might include organizing medical supplies, creating a dedicated space for exercise, or setting up a calming area for relaxation.

- Prioritize changes based on their potential impact on your daily routine and overall well-being. Start with small, manageable adjustments to avoid feeling overwhelmed.

- Implement one change at a time, allowing yourself to adapt before moving on to the next. For example, organize your kitchen to make healthy meal preparation easier.

- Involve family members or housemates in the process. Communicate your needs and encourage them to support your efforts by maintaining the changes.

- Regularly assess the effectiveness of your environment. Make adjustments as needed to ensure it continues to support your self-management goals.

Common pitfalls

- Attempting to make too many changes at once, leading to frustration
- Neglecting to involve others who share your living space

Progress tracking

- Keep a journal of changes made and their impact on your self-management
- Review your environment monthly to identify areas for further improvement

EXERCISE 115. ENGAGING IN RELAXATION ACTIVITIES

Objective

Incorporate relaxation techniques to enhance self-management of chronic diseases

Step-by-step instructions

- Choose a relaxation activity that appeals to you, such as deep breathing, meditation, or gentle yoga. Aim for activities that can be done in 10-15 minutes.

- Set a specific time each day to engage in your chosen relaxation activity. Consistency is key, so try to make it a part of your daily routine.

- Find a quiet, comfortable space where you can focus without distractions. This could be a corner of your living room, a spot in your backyard, or even a quiet room at work.

- Begin your relaxation activity by taking a few deep breaths to center yourself. Focus on your breathing or the movements of your body, depending on the activity.

- If your mind starts to wander, gently bring your focus back to your breathing or the present moment. It's normal for thoughts to arise; the goal is to acknowledge them and return to your relaxation practice.

- After completing the activity, take a moment to notice how you feel. Reflect on any changes in your mood, stress levels, or physical sensations.

- Gradually increase the duration of your relaxation sessions as you become more comfortable with the practice. Aim to reach 20-30 minutes per session over time.

Common pitfalls

- Skipping relaxation activities due to a busy schedule
- Expecting immediate results without giving the practice time to take effect

Progress tracking

- Keep a journal of your relaxation activities, noting the type, duration, and any changes in your well-being
- Review your entries weekly to identify patterns and adjust your routine as needed

EXERCISE 116. PRACTICING GRATITUDE

Objective

Cultivate a positive mindset to enhance self-management of chronic diseases

Step-by-step instructions

- Set aside 5-10 minutes each day for a gratitude practice. Choose a time that fits seamlessly into your routine, such as morning or before bed.

- Find a quiet, comfortable space where you can focus without interruptions. This could be a cozy chair, a spot in your garden, or a peaceful corner of your home.

- Begin by taking a few deep breaths to center yourself. Allow your mind to settle and focus on the present moment.

- Reflect on three things you are grateful for. These can be as simple as a warm cup of coffee, a supportive friend, or a moment of laughter.

- Write down your three gratitude items in a journal or on a piece of paper. Be specific about why each item is meaningful to you.

- If you find it challenging to think of new items, revisit past entries to remind yourself of previous moments of gratitude.

- Over time, aim to expand your gratitude practice by including different aspects of your life, such as health, relationships, or personal achievements.

Common pitfalls

- Struggling to find new items to be grateful for, leading to repetition
- Skipping the practice due to a busy schedule

Progress tracking

- Keep a gratitude journal, noting the date and your three items each day
- Review your entries monthly to observe patterns and shifts in your mindset

EXERCISE 117. VISUALIZING POSITIVE OUTCOMES

Objective

Enhance self-management of chronic diseases by visualizing positive outcomes

Step-by-step instructions

- Set aside 5-10 minutes each day for visualization. Choose a time when you can relax, such as after waking up or before going to bed.

- Find a quiet, comfortable space where you can focus without interruptions. This could be a cozy chair, a spot in your garden, or a peaceful corner of your home.

- Begin by taking a few deep breaths to center yourself. Allow your mind to settle and focus on the present moment.

- Visualize a specific positive outcome related to managing your chronic condition. This could be successfully completing a workout, enjoying a healthy meal, or feeling energetic throughout the day.

- Imagine the details of this positive outcome vividly. Consider the sights, sounds, and feelings associated with achieving this goal.

- If your mind starts to wander, gently bring your focus back to the visualization. It's normal for thoughts to arise; the goal is to acknowledge them and return to your practice.

- After completing the visualization, take a moment to notice how you feel. Reflect on any changes in your mood, motivation, or outlook.

Common pitfalls

- Struggling to visualize specific outcomes, leading to vague or unfocused sessions
- Skipping the practice due to a busy schedule

Progress tracking

- Keep a journal of your visualization sessions, noting the date, the outcome visualized, and any changes in your mindset
- Review your entries monthly to observe patterns and shifts in your motivation

EXERCISE 118. ESTABLISHING A ROUTINE

Objective

Develop a consistent daily routine to enhance self-management
of chronic diseases

Step-by-step instructions

- Identify key daily activities that support your health, such
  as medication intake, meal planning, exercise, and
  relaxation.

- Choose a specific time for each activity, ensuring it fits
  seamlessly into your existing schedule. For example, take
  medication with breakfast or go for a walk after dinner.

- Use a planner or digital calendar to schedule these
  activities, setting reminders to help you stay on track.

- Start with small, manageable changes to avoid feeling
  overwhelmed. Gradually incorporate more activities as
  you become comfortable with your routine.

- Monitor your progress by noting how well you adhere to
  your schedule and any improvements in your symptoms
  or overall well-being.

- Adjust your routine as needed to accommodate changes
  in your lifestyle or health status. Flexibility is key to
  maintaining a sustainable routine.

- Seek support from family or friends to help you stay accountable and motivated.

Common pitfalls

- Overloading your schedule with too many changes at once
- Neglecting to adjust your routine when circumstances change

Progress tracking

- Keep a daily log of your activities and any deviations from your routine
- Review your log weekly to identify patterns and areas for improvement

EXERCISE 119. SEEKING PROFESSIONAL SUPPORT

Objective

Enhance self-management of chronic diseases by effectively seeking and utilizing professional support

Step-by-step instructions

- Identify the type of professional support you need, such as a primary care physician, endocrinologist, dietitian, or physical therapist, based on your specific condition.

- Research and compile a list of potential healthcare providers in your area. Consider factors like location, availability, and patient reviews.

- Verify that the providers on your list accept your insurance plan to minimize out-of-pocket expenses.

- Schedule an appointment with your chosen healthcare provider. Prepare a list of questions and concerns related to your condition to discuss during the visit.

- During the appointment, clearly communicate your symptoms, lifestyle, and any challenges you face in managing your condition. Be honest and open to ensure accurate advice.

- Take notes during the consultation to remember key points and recommendations. Ask for clarification if any advice is unclear.

- Follow up on any referrals or additional tests recommended by your healthcare provider. Schedule these promptly to maintain continuity of care.

- Regularly review your treatment plan with your healthcare provider, especially if there are changes in your symptoms or lifestyle.

Common pitfalls

- Delaying appointments due to busy schedules or financial concerns
- Failing to communicate openly with healthcare providers, leading to incomplete or ineffective treatment plans

Progress tracking

- Keep a record of all healthcare appointments, including dates, providers, and key takeaways
- Review your notes periodically to track improvements and identify areas needing further attention

EXERCISE 120. REFLECTING ON PAST SUCCESSES

Objective

Cultivate a positive mindset by recognizing and building on past
successes in managing chronic diseases

Step-by-step instructions

- Set aside 15 minutes in a quiet space where you can focus
  without distractions.

- Reflect on a specific time when you successfully managed
  a challenging aspect of your chronic condition. This could
  be a day when you maintained your blood sugar levels,
  managed stress effectively, or adhered to your exercise
  routine.

- Write down the details of this success, including what you
  did, how you felt, and the outcome. Be as specific as
  possible to capture the essence of the experience.

- Identify the strategies or actions that contributed to this
  success. Consider factors like planning, support from
  others, or personal motivation.

- Think about how you can apply these strategies to
  current challenges you face in managing your condition.
  Write down at least two ways you can incorporate these
  successful tactics into your daily routine.

- Keep this reflection in a place where you can easily access
  it, such as a journal or a notes app on your phone, to

remind yourself of your capabilities during difficult times.

Common pitfalls

- Focusing only on major successes and overlooking small, everyday achievements
- Allowing negative experiences to overshadow positive reflections

Progress tracking

- Regularly review your reflections to reinforce positive patterns and identify new strategies
- Note any improvements in your mindset or management of your condition as you apply these strategies

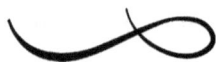

Chapter 21: Nutrition Strategies for Chronic Conditions

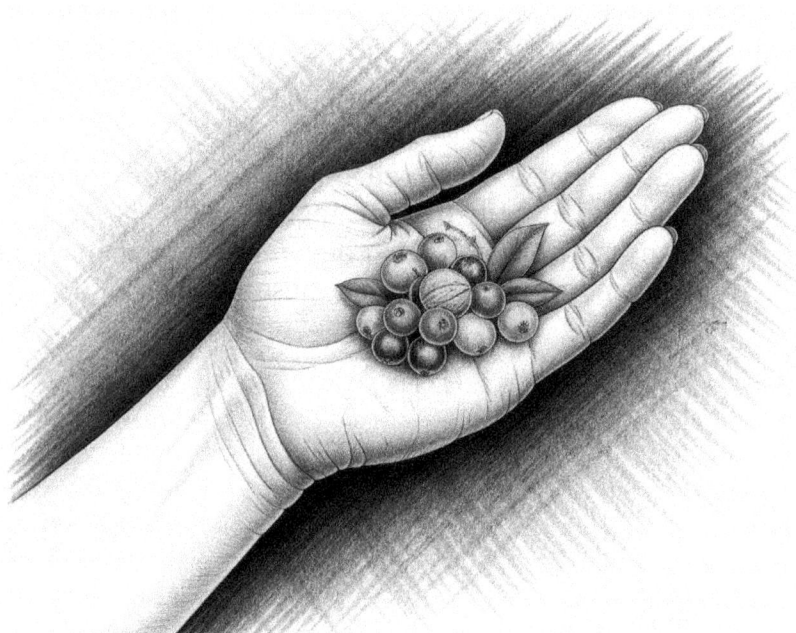

Nutrition plays a vital role in managing chronic diseases like diabetes, hypertension, and musculoskeletal conditions. Embracing a balanced diet centered around whole foods can significantly benefit those facing these health challenges. Whole foods—such as a colorful array of **fruits**, **vegetables**, **lean proteins**, **whole grains**, and **healthy fats**—provide essential nutrients that enhance overall well-being and address specific medical needs.

Carbohydrates, proteins, and fats are the key components of a
healthy diet. Often misunderstood, carbohydrates are crucial for
energy. For individuals with diabetes, closely monitoring
carbohydrate intake is essential for maintaining steady blood
sugar levels. Familiarity with the **glycemic index**, which
indicates how quickly foods can raise blood sugar, can be very
helpful. Opting for foods with a low glycemic index, like:

- whole grains
- legumes
- non-starchy vegetables

can help prevent blood sugar spikes. Additionally, practicing
portion control is important, as it helps manage carbohydrate
consumption at each meal and supports more stable glucose
levels.

Proteins are essential for repairing and maintaining muscles,
particularly for those with musculoskeletal issues. Lean sources
such as chicken, fish, tofu, and legumes provide necessary
amino acids while helping to limit saturated fat intake, which
can be higher in certain animal products. These proteins not
only support muscle health but also help reduce inflammation, a
common concern in musculoskeletal conditions.

Healthy fats from avocados, nuts, seeds, and olive oil are
beneficial for cardiovascular health and managing hypertension.
These fats can lower **LDL cholesterol** and offer anti-

inflammatory benefits that are important for both heart and musculoskeletal health.

Micronutrients, though required in smaller amounts, are equally significant. Individuals with hypertension should be mindful of their sodium intake, as high levels can elevate blood pressure. Choosing fresh, whole foods over processed options can help lower sodium consumption. Incorporating potassium-rich foods like:

- bananas
- sweet potatoes
- spinach

can assist in balancing sodium levels and supporting healthy blood pressure.

Calcium and vitamin D are particularly important for those with musculoskeletal conditions. Foods rich in calcium—such as dairy products, leafy greens, and fortified plant-based milks—are essential for maintaining bone density. Vitamin D, which can be obtained from sunlight and foods like fatty fish and fortified cereals, enhances calcium absorption and supports bone health.

Implementing practical strategies for meal planning and grocery shopping can make it easier to follow these nutritional guidelines. Planning meals in advance allows for thoughtful ingredient choices that align with health goals. Creating a shopping list based on planned meals helps avoid impulse purchases of less nutritious foods. Cooking at home using methods like grilling, steaming, or baking preserves nutrients and minimizes the need for added fats and sodium.

Mindful eating can also enhance dietary habits. This approach encourages individuals to pay close attention during meals, savoring each bite and recognizing hunger and fullness cues. Eating more slowly and focusing on the meal can help foster a healthier relationship with food, leading to better portion control and greater satisfaction.

People managing diabetes should aim for a consistent meal schedule to keep blood sugar levels stable and prevent serious complications like **neuropathy** or **cardiovascular issues**. Dividing daily calories into three main meals and two to three well-timed snacks can help maintain this balance, especially when each meal includes a thoughtful mix of **carbohydrates**, **proteins**, and **healthy fats**. This combination slows glucose absorption and provides sustained energy throughout the day. Utilizing food diaries and mobile apps can be beneficial for tracking carbohydrate intake and monitoring blood glucose, offering valuable insights into how different foods impact levels. This information empowers individuals to make better dietary choices tailored to their unique metabolic responses.

Heart-healthy foods are essential for managing blood pressure in those with hypertension. Consider including the following in your diet:

- Leafy greens like *spinach* and *kale*, which are rich in potassium and help balance sodium.

- Berries such as *blueberries* and *strawberries*, loaded with antioxidants that promote cardiovascular health by reducing oxidative stress.
- Omega-3-rich fish, like *salmon* and *mackerel*, at least twice a week to help lower inflammation and blood pressure.

Reducing processed foods is also crucial, as they often contain excessive sodium and unhealthy trans fats. Instead, consider using herbs and spices like *garlic, basil,* and *turmeric* to enhance flavor while reaping additional health benefits from their anti-inflammatory properties.

Individuals with musculoskeletal conditions can greatly benefit from a diet rich in anti-inflammatory foods, which may alleviate symptoms and enhance joint health. Consider incorporating the following:

- Fatty fish such as *sardines* and *trout*, excellent sources of omega-3 fatty acids known to reduce inflammation and joint pain.
- Nuts and seeds, including *almonds* and *flaxseeds*, which provide essential nutrients and healthy fats that support joint function and mobility.
- Supplements like omega-3 fatty acids and glucosamine; omega-3s can alleviate joint pain and stiffness, while glucosamine supports cartilage health.

Always consult with a healthcare provider before starting any new supplement to ensure it's safe and effective for you.

Understanding nutrition labels is a valuable skill for making informed food choices. Begin by checking the following:

- Serving size and the number of servings per container, as these details influence the total nutritional value.
- Sodium, added sugars, and saturated fats, aiming to keep these low to minimize health risks.
- Foods that are high in dietary fiber, vitamins, and minerals to support overall well-being.

The ingredient list can provide insight into a product's quality; shorter lists with familiar ingredients typically indicate fewer artificial additives.

Setting clear, achievable dietary goals can help maintain motivation and accountability when making changes to eating habits. Identify specific areas for improvement, such as reducing sugar intake or increasing fiber consumption. Break these goals into manageable steps and track your progress regularly. For instance, if your aim is to consume more fiber, start by adding an extra serving of vegetables to one meal each day. Gradually incorporate whole grains and legumes into your diet, and celebrate your progress to encourage continued success.

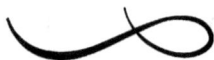

Chapter 22: Safe Exercise and Activity Adaptations

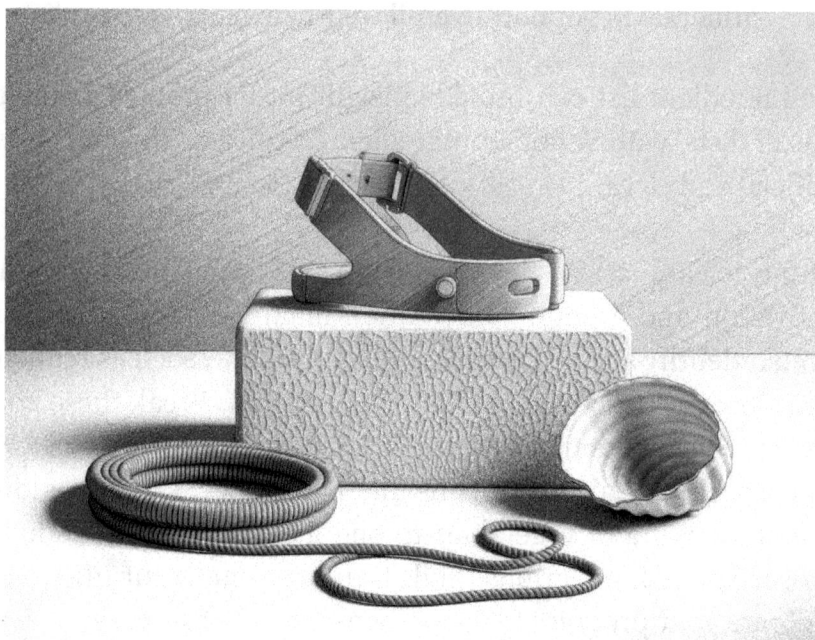

Tip

If you're short on time, try breaking your exercise into several 10-minute sessions throughout the day. Even brief bursts of activity—like a brisk walk during lunch or stretching while watching TV—can add up to real health benefits. Consistency is more important than duration, so focus on making movement a regular part of your routine.

S afe exercise routines are essential for effectively managing chronic conditions like diabetes, hypertension, and musculoskeletal disorders. Engaging in regular physical activity serves as a foundation for overall health management, leading to noticeable improvements in health metrics, enhanced quality of life, and relief from related symptoms. To reap these benefits, it's important to create a personalized plan that aligns with each individual's health status, fitness level, and medical advice.

Starting a safe routine begins with understanding the fundamental principles of physical activity for those with chronic diseases. It's crucial to start slowly, especially for beginners or those returning after a long hiatus. Gradually increasing both intensity and duration helps prevent injuries and allows the body to adapt to new challenges. Being mindful of any discomfort or pain is vital; if negative symptoms arise, they should be addressed promptly, and the plan should be adjusted accordingly.

A personalized exercise strategy should cater to each individual's unique needs and limitations. Consulting healthcare professionals can help identify specific restrictions or recommendations based on medical conditions. For example, individuals with diabetes may need to monitor their *blood glucose* levels before and after exercise, while those with hypertension should steer clear of activities that could lead to sudden spikes in blood pressure. Those dealing with

musculoskeletal issues should focus on exercises that won't
exacerbate joint pain or discomfort.

Different types of activities offer various benefits, so a well-
rounded routine should incorporate a mix of exercises:

- Aerobic activities like walking, swimming, and cycling
  promote cardiovascular health by enhancing heart
  function, circulation, and weight management—key
  elements in managing diabetes and hypertension.
- Strength training is important for building muscle
  support and maintaining bone density, which is
  particularly beneficial for individuals with
  musculoskeletal conditions, as it improves joint stability
  and reduces the risk of injury.
- Flexibility exercises, such as stretching and yoga, help
  maintain joint mobility and prevent stiffness. These
  activities can alleviate discomfort from musculoskeletal
  issues and enhance movement efficiency.
- Balance exercises, including tai chi, are especially
  beneficial for older adults or those facing coordination
  challenges, as they can significantly lower the risk of
  falls—a common concern for individuals with chronic
  health problems.

For those new to exercise or with limited mobility, low-impact
activities are a great option. Walking is accessible and can be
tailored to various fitness levels. Swimming provides a full-body
workout with minimal stress on the joints. Cycling, whether on a
stationary bike or outdoors, offers cardiovascular benefits while
being gentle on the knees and hips. Yoga and tai chi not only
improve flexibility and balance but also promote relaxation and
stress relief, contributing to overall well-being.

People managing diabetes should closely monitor their blood glucose levels around physical activity. This involves checking blood sugar before, during, and after exercise to prevent **hypoglycemia**, which happens when levels drop too low. By keeping a careful eye on these levels, you can take quick action, like having a small carbohydrate-rich snack if your glucose is below 70 mg/dL before starting your workout. It's also essential to choose the right footwear to avoid foot injuries, a common concern due to potential **peripheral neuropathy**. Look for shoes that provide:

- Good arch support
- A comfortable fit without causing friction
- Appropriateness for your activity, whether it's walking, running, or resistance training

Exercises that enhance circulation are particularly beneficial. *Brisk walking* is an excellent option because it's easy to incorporate into most daily routines. **Resistance training** with free weights or resistance bands not only builds muscle strength but also increases **insulin sensitivity**, which helps regulate blood sugar levels. To maximize the benefits, aim to engage in these activities regularly, ideally at least five days a week.

Individuals with hypertension can greatly benefit from moderate-intensity aerobic activities. *Swimming* and *cycling* are especially effective, offering cardiovascular advantages without placing excessive strain on the body. These exercises contribute to lowering blood pressure by enhancing heart function and circulation. It's important to maintain a steady pace and avoid sudden bursts of high-intensity effort, as these can lead to sharp increases in blood pressure. Health guidelines recommend at least 150 minutes of moderate aerobic exercise each week for effective management.

In addition, relaxation techniques play a vital role in managing hypertension. **Deep breathing exercises** and **mindfulness meditation** can significantly reduce stress, a known contributor to high blood pressure. Practicing these techniques daily, even for just five to ten minutes, promotes relaxation and supports heart health. Incorporating them into a cool-down routine after exercise can help gradually lower heart rate and blood pressure.

For those with musculoskeletal issues, exercises that enhance joint flexibility and reduce stiffness are crucial. Gentle stretching routines performed daily can help maintain and improve your range of motion. *Water aerobics* is another excellent choice, as the buoyancy of the water minimizes joint impact while still providing resistance to strengthen muscles. These activities can alleviate discomfort and enhance overall mobility and function.

Physical therapy can be instrumental in creating a personalized exercise plan for individuals facing musculoskeletal challenges. A physical therapist can assess your needs and limitations, then design a program that specifically targets your concerns. This tailored approach ensures that exercises are safe and effective, addressing joint pain, muscle weakness, and balance issues. It's always wise to consult a healthcare provider before starting a new exercise program, especially if you have complex or severe conditions.

Fitting exercise into a busy schedule while managing chronic conditions requires a thoughtful and personalized approach. Begin by setting clear, measurable goals that resonate with your lifestyle and health needs. Break these objectives into manageable steps, such as aiming for several **10-minute** activity sessions throughout the day. This strategy not only makes physical activity more achievable but also helps maintain your energy levels and reduce fatigue.

Having a structured schedule is essential. Identify specific times in your daily routine to incorporate short bursts of activity. For instance, consider taking a brisk **10-minute** walk during lunch or doing a quick set of bodyweight exercises while waiting for your coffee. These small, consistent efforts can accumulate and have a significant positive impact on your fitness and overall well-being.

Technology can be a great ally in keeping you motivated and tracking your progress. Fitness trackers and mobile apps can:

- Count your steps
- Monitor your heart rate
- Send reminders to move

These features are especially helpful for those managing chronic conditions. These tools provide instant feedback, helping you stay accountable and adjust your routine as needed. Many apps also offer community features, allowing you to connect with others who share similar health goals and build a supportive network.

Choosing activities you genuinely enjoy is key to maintaining an exercise routine. Whether it's *dancing*, *hiking*, or joining a local sports team, selecting something fun makes it easier to stay committed over time. Inviting friends or family to join can enhance the social aspect of your workouts, making them more enjoyable. Group activities not only boost motivation but also create a support system that helps you navigate challenges.

Common barriers like limited time, low motivation, or fear of injury can be addressed with creative solutions. Incorporate movement into your day by:

- Taking the stairs instead of the elevator
- Parking farther away
- Using a standing desk

Home workouts, such as bodyweight routines or online fitness classes, offer convenience and flexibility, allowing you to exercise at your own pace and comfort level.

Self-care and rest are crucial components of any exercise plan, especially when managing chronic conditions. Listen to your body and schedule recovery time to prevent burnout and minimize the risk of injury. Plan rest days and include activities that promote relaxation, like stretching or meditation. These practices support both physical recovery and mental well-being, which are vital for maintaining your motivation.

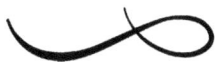

Chapter 23: Home Health Monitoring and Progress Tracking

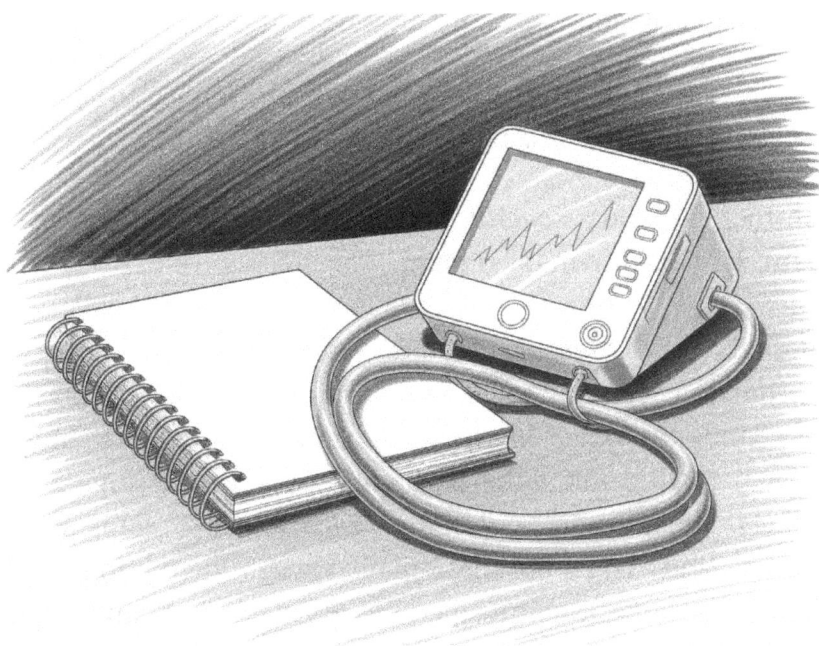

Regular health monitoring at home is vital for individuals managing chronic conditions like **diabetes**, **hypertension**, and **musculoskeletal disorders**. By consistently tracking key health metrics—such as blood pressure readings, blood glucose levels, weight, and physical activity—you gain valuable insights into how well your self-management strategies are working and can spot potential complications early. This proactive approach empowers you to take control of your health and enhances your ability to share accurate data with healthcare providers, leading to more personalized and effective care.

A home health monitoring toolkit is the cornerstone of this strategy. It includes simple, cost-effective tools that are easy to use and provide essential data for managing chronic diseases. The main components consist of:

- A digital blood pressure monitor
- A glucometer
- A weight scale
- A pedometer or fitness tracker

Each tool measures specific health parameters that are crucial for effective disease management.

A digital blood pressure monitor is essential for those with hypertension. It allows for regular checks of blood pressure levels and provides immediate feedback on how lifestyle changes, medication adherence, or stress levels impact your readings. Keeping a systematic record helps you identify patterns and triggers that may cause fluctuations. This information supports informed health decisions, and regular monitoring can alert you to potential issues, such as consistently high readings that may need medical attention.

For diabetes management, a glucometer measures blood glucose levels and shows how your dietary choices, physical activity, and medication regimens affect your control. Regular checks help you understand how your body responds to different foods and activities, making it easier to adjust your management strategies promptly. Maintaining a detailed log of glucose levels also fosters collaboration with healthcare providers to refine treatment plans and prevent complications like *neuropathy* or *cardiovascular diseases.*

A weight scale is another important component of the home health monitoring toolkit. Tracking your weight is crucial for those with chronic conditions, as fluctuations can significantly impact management. For instance, weight gain can worsen hypertension and increase the risk of complications in diabetes, while weight loss can enhance blood pressure regulation and improve insulin sensitivity. Consistent monitoring allows you to evaluate the effectiveness of dietary and exercise interventions and make necessary adjustments to achieve your health goals.

A pedometer or fitness tracker offers valuable insights into your physical activity levels. Regular exercise is key to managing chronic diseases, and tracking your steps or duration can motivate you to stay active. These devices help you set realistic activity goals and monitor your progress over time. Reviewing your activity patterns can uncover opportunities to increase physical activity, supporting better health outcomes.

Each of these tools plays a crucial role in chronic disease management by providing data that informs your self-management decisions. The greatest benefits arise when they are used together, offering a comprehensive overview of your health. Combining data from multiple sources gives you a holistic understanding of your health status and supports more informed decisions about your care, strengthening disease management and encouraging active participation in maintaining your health.

To use a digital blood pressure monitor correctly, start by selecting a cuff that fits your arm circumference; using the wrong size can lead to inaccurate readings. Sit comfortably in a chair with your back supported and your feet flat on the floor for stability. Rest your arm on a table at heart level and wrap the cuff around your upper arm, about an inch above the elbow crease. Take a moment to remain still and quiet for at least five minutes before taking a measurement, allowing your cardiovascular system to settle into a resting state. When you're ready, press the **start** button and maintain your position as the cuff inflates and deflates. The monitor will display two important numbers: **systolic pressure**, which measures the force of blood against artery walls during heartbeats, and **diastolic pressure**, which indicates the pressure when the heart relaxes between beats. It's a good idea to record these values in a health journal or digital app to track trends and support discussions with your healthcare provider.

People managing diabetes rely on a glucometer for daily health checks. Start by washing your hands with warm water to remove contaminants and improve blood flow. Insert a test strip into the device, ensuring it's positioned correctly for accurate results. Use a lancet device to prick the side of your fingertip, which is less sensitive than the pad, and gently squeeze to produce a drop of blood. Touch the test strip to the droplet, and the glucometer will display your blood sugar level within seconds. Checking glucose at different times—such as fasting in the morning and two hours after meals—helps you understand your body's patterns. Keeping a consistent log of these readings makes it easier to spot trends and adjust your diet or medication as needed.

Consistency is key when tracking weight. Use a digital scale and weigh yourself at the same time each day, preferably in the morning after using the restroom and before eating or drinking. Wear minimal clothing for more accurate results, and place the scale on a hard, flat surface to avoid errors from uneven flooring. Regular tracking provides valuable feedback on how well your diet and exercise plans are working and can motivate you to maintain or adjust your approach as necessary.

Fitness trackers help monitor physical activity and set achievable goals. Set a daily step target that matches your current fitness level, and gradually increase it as your endurance builds. Most devices also display **heart rate** and **calories burned**, giving you a clear picture of your activity levels. Use this information to tailor your exercise routine and balance aerobic, strength, and flexibility training. Many trackers sync with mobile apps, allowing you to log activities and spot trends over time. Reviewing this data can highlight periods of inactivity and encourage you to add more movement to your day.

Reviewing the health data collected at home is essential for effectively managing chronic conditions. Make it a regular practice to examine your records each week to identify trends and patterns. For instance, if your blood pressure readings frequently exceed **130/80 mmHg** in the evenings, it may be time to rethink your evening routine or adjust your medication schedule. Similarly, if blood glucose levels consistently rise above **180 mg/dL** after certain meals, consider reassessing your diet. Recognizing these patterns empowers you to make informed choices about lifestyle adjustments or to have meaningful discussions with your healthcare provider.

Setting clear, measurable health goals is a great way to enhance disease control. Use your baseline data to create realistic and specific targets. For example, if your average blood pressure is **140/90 mmHg**, aim to lower it to **126/82 mmHg** over the next three months, which represents about a 10% reduction. If your blood sugar levels often exceed the target range of **70-130 mg/dL**, strive to keep them within this range at least **80%** of the time. Tailor these goals to your personal health needs and review them with your healthcare provider to ensure they are both safe and achievable.

Knowing when to make changes is crucial for effective condition management. If your blood pressure readings remain above **140/90 mmHg** despite following your treatment plan, don't hesitate to reach out to your healthcare provider to discuss potential medication adjustments or new lifestyle strategies. If your blood glucose levels fluctuate significantly, this may indicate a need to modify your diet or reassess your insulin plan. Taking proactive steps when these issues arise can help prevent complications and enhance your overall health.

Bringing your tracked data to regular check-ups allows healthcare providers to offer personalized feedback and recommendations. Whether you use digital records or printed copies, sharing this information during appointments fosters more comprehensive discussions about your progress and any concerns. Providers can review your data, suggest modifications to treatment plans, and provide guidance on achieving your health goals. Collaborating in this manner ensures that management strategies are tailored to your specific needs and circumstances.

Staying motivated over the long term can be challenging, but certain strategies can help you maintain your momentum. Celebrating milestones, such as reaching a target blood pressure of **120/80 mmHg** or keeping your blood glucose within the desired range for a month, can boost your motivation and reinforce healthy habits. Involving family members in your health goals adds an extra layer of support and accountability. Share your objectives with loved ones and invite them to participate in healthy activities, like preparing nutritious meals or going for walks together.

Online communities can offer additional encouragement and support. Many platforms feature forums where individuals with similar conditions share experiences, provide tips, and motivate one another. Connecting with these groups can alleviate feelings of isolation and offer valuable insights for managing your conditions. These communities often celebrate collective achievements, fostering a sense of camaraderie and shared purpose.

Tools for Tracking Symptoms, Medications, and Progress

In today's fast-paced world, managing chronic diseases like **diabetes**, **hypertension**, and **musculoskeletal disorders** calls for a thoughtful approach. This means keeping an eye on symptoms, sticking to medication schedules, and tracking progress toward specific health goals. A range of practical tools and techniques can support individuals in this journey, from innovative digital solutions to tried-and-true traditional methods.

Digital tools have revolutionized health management, making it more convenient and precise. Smartphone applications and online platforms now offer features designed to meet the unique needs of those with chronic conditions. Many of these apps include symptom logging, allowing users to record daily health changes, such as:

- Blood sugar levels
- Blood pressure readings
- Joint pain intensity on a numerical scale

Maintaining a digital log helps individuals spot patterns and potential triggers, which can lead to more productive conversations with healthcare providers.

Sticking to prescribed medication is vital for managing chronic diseases. Digital solutions cater to this need with various applications that provide customizable reminders, helping users take their doses on time. These notifications can be tailored to fit each person's routine, significantly reducing the chance of missed doses and leading to improved treatment outcomes. Some platforms also allow users to track medication side effects, offering a more complete picture of how different treatments impact daily life.

Tracking health goals is another essential feature found in many digital tools. Users can set specific targets, such as reaching a certain blood pressure or maintaining a particular level of physical activity. These platforms often include progress tracking, enabling individuals to see their achievements over time. Visualizing progress through graphs or charts can help maintain motivation and facilitate adjustments to management strategies when needed.

Wearable technology, like smartwatches and fitness trackers, complements digital tools by providing real-time data on vital signs, physical activity, and sleep patterns. These devices use sensors to monitor:

- Heart rate
- Step count
- Sleep quality

Individuals managing hypertension can gain insights into how daily activities affect blood pressure through continuous heart rate monitoring. Those with diabetes can benefit from tracking physical activity, as regular exercise is crucial for controlling blood sugar.

Connecting wearable technology with smartphone applications enhances the user experience by syncing data automatically. This integration offers a holistic view of health metrics and supports informed decisions. For instance, if a smartwatch detects a sudden increase in heart rate, the user might check their blood pressure and take action if necessary.

While digital tools offer numerous benefits, traditional methods still hold value for those who prefer a hands-on approach. Health journals or notebooks provide a tangible way to track symptoms, medication use, and significant health changes. Writing down daily observations can be therapeutic, helping individuals process their experiences and stay engaged in managing their health.

Keeping a consistent record in a health journal aids in identifying trends and triggers. For example, noting when joint pain begins after certain activities can help those with musculoskeletal issues adjust their routines to minimize discomfort. Recording meals alongside blood sugar readings can assist individuals with diabetes in pinpointing which foods lead to glucose spikes.

Choosing between digital and traditional tools ultimately depends on personal preference and lifestyle. Some appreciate the speed and convenience of digital solutions, while others enjoy the tactile experience of writing in a journal. Regardless of the method chosen, **consistency** is key. Regular tracking, whether digital or manual, provides valuable insights that empower individuals to take charge of their health.

To make the most of digital applications for managing chronic diseases, begin by selecting one that aligns with your specific health needs. There are many options available to help you monitor symptoms, medication schedules, and health goals. After choosing an app, enter essential details like your age, weight, and diagnosed conditions. This information enables the software to customize its features to suit your situation.

Set up alerts and notifications that work for you. For medication tracking, input prescription details, including dosages and timing. Schedule reminders that fit seamlessly into your daily routine, ensuring you receive notifications when necessary. This strategy helps you stick to your treatment plan and reduces the likelihood of missing doses. Some applications also allow you to log side effects or adverse reactions, giving you a more comprehensive view of how medications impact you each day.

Utilize the app to track symptoms by recording daily changes in your health, such as:

- Blood sugar levels
- Blood pressure
- Pain intensity

Many apps present this information in graphs or charts, making it easier to identify trends over time. These visual tools help you understand how factors like diet and physical activity influence your condition. Regularly reviewing these trends can guide adjustments to your management plan and foster more productive conversations with your healthcare provider.

Smartwatches and fitness trackers provide real-time monitoring of vital signs and activity levels. To get the most out of these devices, connect them to your chosen health app. This setup allows for automatic data transfer and offers a complete view of your health metrics. Continuous heart rate monitoring, for instance, can reveal how stress or exercise impacts cardiovascular health. Tracking steps and activity levels can inspire you to achieve your exercise goals, which is crucial for managing conditions like **diabetes** and **hypertension**.

Understanding data from wearable devices is key to interpreting health trends. Heart rate patterns can provide insights into cardiovascular fitness and stress levels. If your resting heart rate remains elevated, it might be a good time to increase physical activity or focus on stress management. Activity levels, measured in steps or active minutes, indicate how much you move each day. Gradually working to improve these numbers can lead to better health outcomes.

If you prefer to track your health manually, use a structured format to organize your daily observations. Keeping a health journal or notebook can help you record symptoms, medication doses, and adherence to your treatment plan. Create a daily log with sections for each aspect of health management, such as:

- Morning and evening blood pressure readings
- Blood sugar levels before and after meals
- Any symptoms you notice throughout the day

Set aside time each week to review your recorded data. Going over your logs helps you identify patterns and measure progress toward your health goals. This practice can reveal areas where you might need to make adjustments, like modifying your diet or exercise routine. Sharing these insights with your healthcare provider can lead to more personalized and effective treatment plans.

Tracking symptoms and medications daily can greatly enhance the management of chronic conditions. Choose a specific time, like **7:00 AM** or **9:00 PM**, to update your health logs and review your progress. Sticking to this schedule helps ensure accuracy and consistency. Incorporate this step into your morning routine or just before bed, when things are usually quieter, allowing for focused reflection without interruptions. Treating this as a daily habit makes it second nature—much like brushing your teeth or savoring your morning coffee.

Charts and graphs offer a straightforward way to monitor trends and pinpoint areas that need attention. These visual tools make it easier to notice patterns or changes in your health over time. For example, a line graph of blood pressure readings for the past month can quickly highlight any upward trends that may need action. A bar chart tracking blood sugar levels can reveal which meals or activities lead to spikes or drops, helping you make informed dietary or exercise adjustments.

Having an **accountability partner** can boost your commitment to tracking habits and achieving health goals. Involve family members or friends in your health management for added encouragement and motivation. Share your objectives with them and ask for their help in reminding you to update logs or take medications. This shared responsibility fosters commitment and creates a sense of support, making the process feel less isolating.

To address common challenges like forgetfulness or low motivation, plan ahead and use habit-building strategies. Set reminders on your phone or utilize a health tracking app to ensure you don't miss important updates. Schedule these reminders for the same time each day to align with your routine. You can also try *habit-stacking*—pairing a new habit with an existing one. For instance, if you always drink a glass of water in the morning, use that moment to update your health log as well.

Recognizing small achievements keeps you engaged and committed to health management. Reward yourself for reaching milestones, such as logging symptoms for **30 consecutive days** or achieving a target blood pressure of **120/80 mmHg**. Even simple rewards, like enjoying a favorite activity or a special meal, can reinforce your progress and maintain motivation.

Periodically review your tracking methods and make adjustments if something isn't working effectively. If a particular tool or technique isn't yielding the desired results, explore different approaches. The goal is to find a system that fits seamlessly into your life and supports your health objectives. Flexibility and adaptability are key, allowing for adjustments as your conditions or routines change.

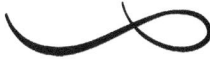

Chapter 24: Preventing Complications and Flare-Ups

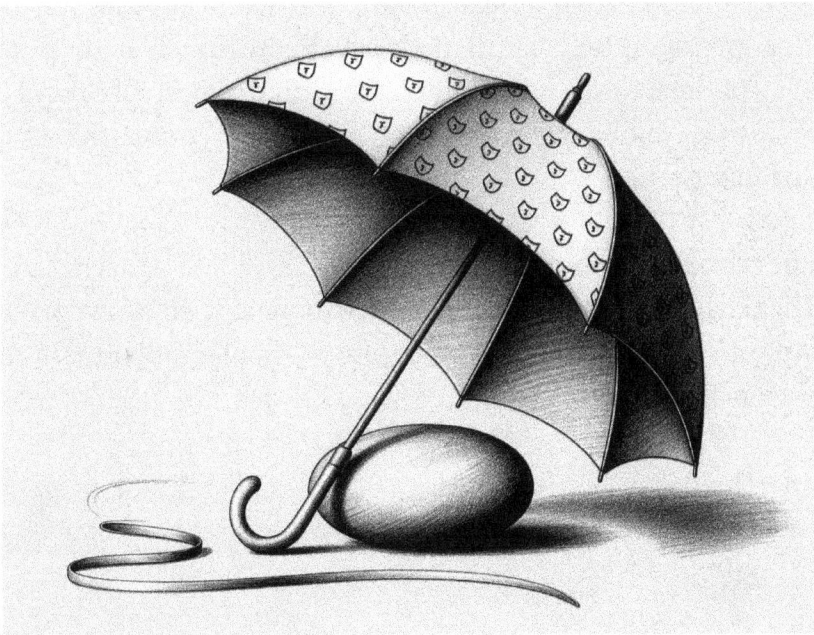

Spotting early warning signs of complications and flare-ups in chronic diseases is essential for effectively managing and preventing serious health issues. Individuals living with conditions like **diabetes**, **hypertension**, and **musculoskeletal disorders** can greatly benefit from being attentive to subtle changes in their health. This awareness not only helps maintain stability but also plays a crucial role in avoiding more severe episodes.

In **diabetes**, complications may first show up as unusual fatigue, frequent urination, increased thirst, or unexpected weight loss. These symptoms often indicate shifts in blood sugar levels that, if not addressed, can lead to serious problems such as **neuropathy** or **cardiovascular disease**. Responses can vary widely; for instance, a slight rise in blood sugar might leave one person feeling significantly fatigued, while another may not notice any symptoms until their levels are much higher. This range of reactions highlights the importance of regularly monitoring blood glucose and tailoring assessments to individual needs.

Hypertension, often referred to as the "silent killer," can be particularly challenging because it typically doesn't present symptoms until it becomes dangerous. Some individuals may experience:

- Headaches
- Shortness of breath
- Nosebleeds

These signs can signal the need for further evaluation, even though they aren't exclusive to high blood pressure. Regularly checking blood pressure reveals how lifestyle choices and stress impact cardiovascular health. Recognizing patterns, such as consistently high readings, allows for timely action to prevent complications like heart disease or stroke.

Musculoskeletal disorders, such as arthritis and chronic back pain, often manifest early as joint stiffness, swelling, or ongoing discomfort. These symptoms can fluctuate based on activity levels, weather, or stress. Being mindful of how your body typically reacts to different situations can help you anticipate when a flare-up might occur. For example, if you notice increased stiffness after sitting for long periods, it may be a good idea to incorporate more movement into your daily routine to alleviate discomfort.

Triggers for these symptoms can be diverse and complex. Diet plays a significant role in managing chronic conditions; for instance, high-sugar foods can lead to blood glucose spikes in diabetes, while excessive sodium can worsen hypertension. A lack of physical activity often results in weight gain, higher blood pressure, and stiffer joints. Additionally, stress—both physical and emotional—can have a considerable impact on health, sometimes raising blood pressure or intensifying musculoskeletal pain.

Environmental factors, such as changes in weather or exposure to allergens, can also influence the severity of symptoms. Cold weather may exacerbate joint pain for those with arthritis, and high pollen counts can aggravate respiratory issues in individuals with hypertension. Staying aware of these triggers and their effects on your body can help you manage your condition more effectively.

Being attentive to your body's signals is vital. Regularly checking your health and noting any changes from your usual patterns can make a significant difference. Keeping a health journal is a practical way to track symptoms, identify possible triggers, and observe trends over time. This approach not only aids in catching complications early but also provides the information needed to make informed choices about your health.

Recognizing early signs of complications requires prompt and informed action to prevent further issues. Begin with a thorough assessment of the situation and pinpoint any potential triggers. For example, if you notice a sudden increase in blood pressure, consider making dietary adjustments, such as lowering sodium intake to below **2,300 mg** per day, and incorporating light physical activity like a brisk **10-minute walk** to help bring it down. When managing diabetes, a spike in blood glucose levels calls for a careful review of recent meals to identify any dietary missteps. Taking corrective steps, such as ensuring your next meal includes at least **15 grams of fiber** and a source of **lean protein**, can help stabilize your sugar levels.

Reaching out to healthcare providers is crucial when early signs of complications arise. Contact your primary care physician or a nurse practitioner to discuss your symptoms and receive tailored advice. They may recommend temporary adjustments to your medication regimen, such as changing dosages or switching medications, or suggest further tests like blood work or imaging studies to gain a clearer understanding of your condition. Always adhere to medical guidance before making any changes to your treatment plan, as self-modification without professional input can lead to unintended health consequences.

Creating a personalized action plan is key to effectively managing potential flare-ups. This plan should include a comprehensive list of emergency contacts, such as:

- Your primary care physician
- A trusted family member
- Any specialists involved in your care

Keep an updated list of all medications, including specific dosages and administration schedules, in a place that's easy to access. Clearly outline the steps to take in case of a flare-up, such as using a prescribed rescue medication or practicing a specific relaxation technique like *progressive muscle relaxation* to manage stress-induced symptoms.

Ongoing management of chronic conditions relies on regular communication with healthcare professionals. Schedule routine check-ins, ideally every three to six months, to review symptoms and discuss any changes in your health status. These appointments provide an opportunity to adjust your management plan, ensuring it remains effective and aligned with your current needs. Maintaining an open dialogue with your healthcare team fosters a collaborative approach to care and empowers you to make informed decisions about your health.

Managing stress is vital in preventing the worsening of symptoms. Mindfulness practices, such as deep breathing exercises or guided meditation, can significantly reduce stress levels when incorporated into your daily routine. These

techniques are particularly beneficial for conditions like
hypertension, where stress can elevate blood pressure. Engaging
in activities that promote relaxation, such as *yoga* or *tai chi*,
also enhances both physical flexibility and mental clarity.

Having a supportive network is invaluable for managing chronic
diseases. Connect with community resources or support groups
to meet others who share similar experiences. These groups
offer a space to exchange practical tips, discuss challenges, and
provide mutual encouragement. The camaraderie and
understanding found in these communities can inspire you to
stay committed to your health goals.

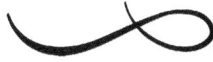

Chapter 25: Managing Chronic Disease at Work and Home

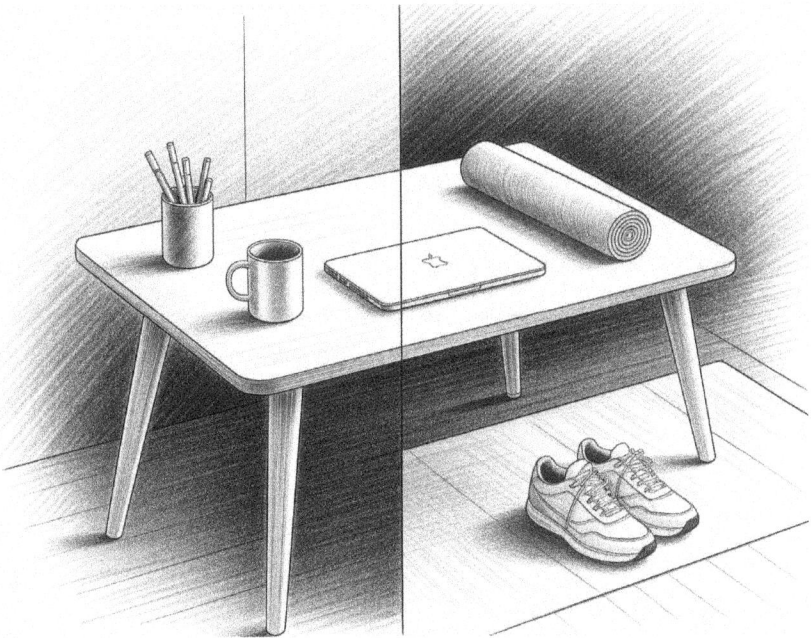

Managing chronic conditions like **diabetes**, **hypertension**, and **musculoskeletal disorders** calls for a structured approach that seamlessly fits into your daily routines at work and home. Establishing effective health management routines is essential for maintaining good health and preventing complications. By incorporating medication schedules, meal planning, and exercise regimens into your daily life, you create a solid foundation for managing your well-being.

Begin with a daily schedule tailored to your specific health needs. For those with diabetes, this might mean setting specific times for blood glucose checks, such as before meals and at bedtime, along with regular insulin doses. If you're managing hypertension, monitoring your blood pressure at the same times each day and sticking closely to prescribed medications is crucial. Individuals with musculoskeletal disorders can benefit from integrating specific physical therapy exercises or stretching routines into their day, which can help alleviate discomfort and improve mobility. This approach ensures that the most important aspects of each condition are effectively addressed.

A balanced work-life schedule is vital for reducing fatigue and preventing burnout. Make sure to allocate time for physical activity, which benefits all chronic conditions. This could include:

- A brisk 30-minute walk during lunch
- A 20-minute workout before your day starts
- Regular exercise to support weight management, lower stress, and promote heart health

Incorporating stress-reducing techniques like deep breathing or short meditation sessions can also enhance your mental well-being. Prioritizing rest is equally important; aim for 7-9 hours of quality sleep each night to support overall health and recovery.

Organizational tools can make managing chronic diseases much simpler. Use planners or digital apps to track symptoms, medication times, and medical appointments. Many health management apps offer reminders and alerts to help you stay on top of your doses and follow-up visits. Keeping a detailed record of health metrics can help you identify trends and make informed choices about your care. This proactive approach not only facilitates effective management but also leads to more productive conversations with healthcare providers.

Creating a home environment that supports health management is also essential. Store medications and health-monitoring devices in a specific, easily accessible location to help maintain your routine. For those with musculoskeletal issues, ergonomic furniture or supportive cushions can enhance comfort and reduce strain. A well-organized space can lower stress and simplify daily health tasks.

At work, good ergonomics can minimize physical strain and boost productivity. Arrange your desk to promote good posture, ensuring your computer screen is at eye level and your chair supports your lower back. Remember to take regular breaks— stand, stretch, or walk for a few minutes every hour to prevent stiffness and improve circulation. These small adjustments can significantly impact managing musculoskeletal discomfort and maintaining focus throughout the day.

Setting realistic goals and priorities is key to balancing productivity with health management. Break tasks into smaller steps to make progress without feeling overwhelmed. This method enhances efficiency and allows you to protect your health while achieving work objectives. By concentrating on priorities and establishing achievable goals, you can feel accomplished and keep your well-being at the forefront.

Effective communication is essential for managing chronic conditions, both at home and in the workplace. Establishing clear and open channels with family members is key to understanding your specific health needs and ensuring you receive the support you require. Begin by sharing detailed information about your condition, including:

- Descriptions of symptoms
- Treatment plans
- Any lifestyle changes, such as dietary adjustments or exercise routines

This approach helps your loved ones understand the challenges you face and fosters a supportive environment. Encourage them to ask questions and share their concerns, creating a dialogue that enhances mutual understanding and cooperation.

At work, discussing your situation with colleagues can cultivate a more supportive and accommodating atmosphere. Have a conversation with your supervisor or human resources department about your health needs, emphasizing any accommodations you may require, such as:

- Flexible hours
- Remote work options
- Ergonomic adjustments to your workspace

When appropriate, share relevant information with close colleagues so they can better understand your circumstances and find ways to support you. This openness helps prevent misunderstandings and promotes empathy and collaboration.

Regular appointments with healthcare providers are vital for monitoring your condition and updating treatment plans as necessary. Schedule routine check-ins to review your progress, discuss any changes in symptoms, and consider potential adjustments to your management strategy. These meetings provide a structured opportunity to address concerns and receive professional advice, ensuring your treatment remains effective and aligned with your current health status. Keeping a detailed log of symptoms and health metrics, such as **blood pressure** or **glucose levels**, can enhance these discussions and support informed decision-making.

Assertive communication techniques are valuable for expressing your needs and boundaries effectively in both personal and professional settings. Use clear and direct language, relying on *"I"* statements to convey your feelings and requirements without placing blame or causing defensiveness. For instance, say, *"I need to take a break every hour to manage my condition,"* instead of, *"You never let me take breaks."* This approach encourages understanding and respect, making it easier to advocate for your health needs.

Encouraging participation in family or workplace wellness programs can enhance collective health awareness and strengthen mutual support. These initiatives often provide resources and activities that benefit everyone, such as:

- Fitness challenges

- Nutrition workshops
- Stress management seminars

Involving family or colleagues in these programs fosters a shared commitment to health and well-being, which can boost motivation and accountability.

Leveraging technology can help maintain communication with healthcare teams. Telehealth services and messaging apps offer convenient ways to stay connected with providers, making it easier to receive timely updates and interventions when needed. These tools allow you to share health data, ask questions, and receive advice without the need for in-person visits, which is especially beneficial for busy schedules. Make sure you have the necessary apps and devices set up, and take some time to learn how they work to maximize their benefits.

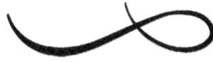

Chapter 26: Building a Supportive Healthcare Team

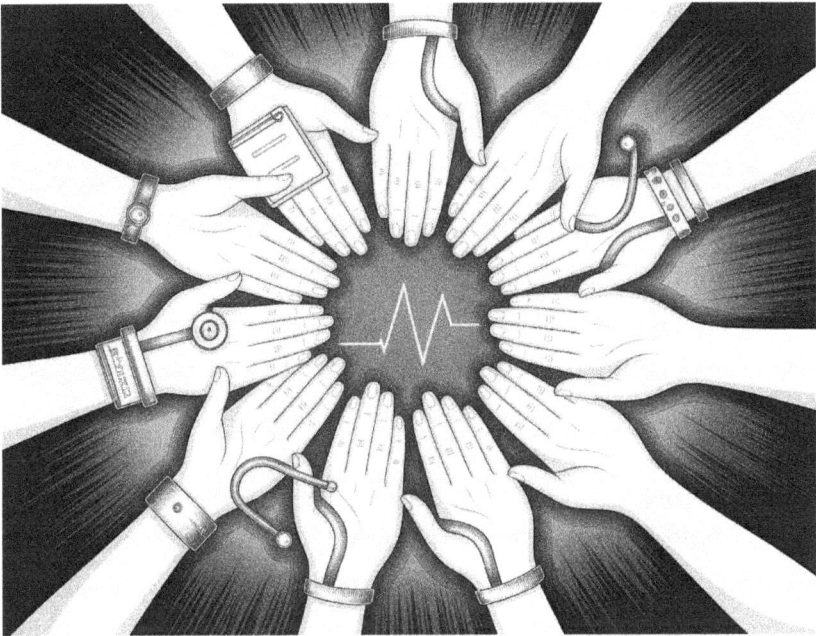

Tip

Before each medical appointment, prepare a written list of your questions, symptoms, and any recent changes in your health. Prioritize your most pressing concerns at the top. This simple step helps you make the most of your limited time with providers, ensures nothing important is

*forgotten, and empowers you to take an active role in your
care. Being organized also helps your healthcare team
address your needs more efficiently, leading to better
outcomes.*

C reating a supportive healthcare team is essential for
effectively managing chronic diseases like diabetes,
hypertension, and musculoskeletal
disorders. The first step is to identify and select the right
professionals who can provide care tailored to your unique
needs. This process involves understanding the roles of various
specialists and how each can contribute to your overall health
management.

Start your search by exploring the types of healthcare providers
that are key to managing chronic conditions. A **primary care
physician (PCP)** typically serves as your main point of
contact, coordinating care, monitoring your health, and
referring you to specialists when necessary. For diabetes, an
endocrinologist brings expertise in hormonal regulation,
helping you manage blood sugar levels and insulin therapy. If
you're dealing with hypertension, a **cardiologist** can offer
specialized care for cardiovascular health and related
complications. For musculoskeletal issues, an **orthopedic
specialist** or **rheumatologist** can diagnose and treat joint
and muscle disorders.

Consider adding a **registered dietitian** to your team. They can
provide personalized nutritional assessments and dietary plans
that support your condition through targeted nutrition.

Physical therapists are also valuable, especially for musculoskeletal concerns, as they design exercise regimens to enhance mobility and alleviate pain.

Once you've identified the types of professionals you need, evaluate potential providers by looking for those with a strong track record in treating your specific condition. Review their experience, qualifications, and board certifications. Patient reviews and testimonials can offer insight into their reputation and the quality of care they provide. It's important to assess how they approach patient care:

- Do they listen to your concerns?
- Are they open to discussing different treatment options and collaborating with other members of your healthcare team?
- How do they communicate information?

Pay attention to communication style. Choose providers who explain information clearly and ensure you understand your condition and treatment plan. They should be approachable and responsive, creating an environment where you feel comfortable discussing your health.

Set up initial consultations with potential providers to see if they are a good fit for your needs. Prepare questions that help you understand their treatment philosophy and availability. Ask how they integrate lifestyle changes with medical treatment, as this approach is often key to managing chronic diseases. Inquire about their availability for appointments and follow-up care procedures.

Logistics matter as well. Check the location of their clinics and whether they offer **telehealth services**, which can make accessing care easier without frequent in-person visits. Ensure the providers you choose are in-network with your insurance plan to avoid unexpected costs and keep healthcare affordable.

Open and honest communication with every member of your healthcare team is essential for effectively managing chronic conditions. Share detailed information about your symptoms, daily routines, lifestyle choices, and personal health goals. This comprehensive background helps create treatment plans tailored to your specific needs. For instance, if you have **diabetes**, providing insights into your daily schedule, eating habits, and activity levels allows your endocrinologist to adjust your insulin dosage or recommend dietary changes that suit you best.

Keep your providers informed whenever your condition changes. Letting the team know about new symptoms, medication side effects, or challenges with your regimen enables timely adjustments to your treatment. For example, if you start feeling dizzy after beginning a new **hypertension** medication, informing your doctor right away allows them to modify the dosage or explore alternative options, minimizing the risk of complications.

Building mutual trust with healthcare professionals is crucial for managing chronic diseases. Take an active role in your treatment by asking specific questions and seeking clarification on medical advice. This approach enhances your understanding of your health and empowers you to make informed decisions.

For example, if your rheumatologist suggests a new therapy for **arthritis**, ask about its benefits, potential side effects, and how it fits into your overall care plan. These conversations foster a partnership where you feel confident in the care you receive.

Request feedback on your progress to strengthen your relationship with providers. Regularly seek their input on health improvements and discuss areas that may need more attention. This practice helps you stay aligned with your health goals and demonstrates your commitment to managing your condition. Expressing gratitude to your team for their support and guidance also nurtures a positive, collaborative partnership. Even a simple acknowledgment of their efforts can significantly enhance your connection.

A team-based approach is vital for comprehensive care. Help various healthcare providers stay connected by sharing your medical records and updates. This coordination ensures everyone is on the same page, reducing the likelihood of conflicting advice or unnecessary tests. For example, if your cardiologist prescribes a new medication, make sure your primary care doctor and other specialists are informed. Keeping everyone updated leads to a more cohesive treatment plan that addresses all aspects of your health.

Leverage technology to enhance communication and information sharing. Many healthcare systems offer patient portals where you can access your medical records, view test results, and message your providers. These tools keep everyone involved in your care informed and facilitate better coordination. You can also use apps to track symptoms, medication schedules, and lifestyle changes. Sharing this information with your healthcare team provides them with a clearer picture of your health and supports more effective decision-making.

Active listening is essential for effective communication with healthcare providers. It's about giving your full attention to the speaker, truly absorbing what they say rather than just hearing the words. To enhance this skill, focus on the person speaking, maintain steady eye contact, and avoid interruptions. After receiving advice or instructions, repeating the information back can help confirm your understanding. For instance, if your doctor explains a new medication schedule, you might say, "Just to confirm, I should take this pill twice daily, once in the morning and once in the evening, right?" This approach not only checks your understanding but also invites any necessary clarification.

Clear and direct communication is crucial when discussing your health. When describing symptoms or concerns, use specific examples to create a vivid picture. Instead of saying, "I feel unwell," you could say, "I've been experiencing **sharp pain** in my lower back for the past three days, especially when I stand up after sitting." Stick to language you're comfortable with, and if a medical term comes up that you don't understand, don't hesitate to ask your provider to explain it in simpler terms to avoid any confusion.

Preparing ahead of time can help you maximize your medical appointments. Before each visit, jot down a detailed list of questions, symptoms, and any recent changes in your health.

Prioritize the most important items at the top so you can address them first. For example, if you've noticed a new side effect from a medication, make sure to bring it up early in your conversation with your doctor. Having a written list keeps you organized and ensures you cover all your concerns during the appointment.

Assertive communication empowers you to express your needs and preferences clearly. Be honest about what you can realistically manage regarding treatment plans and mention any challenges you face. If a prescribed exercise routine feels too difficult, let your healthcare provider know by saying, "I understand the importance of exercise, but the current plan is too intense for me. Can we adjust it to better fit my capabilities?" This way, your input is valued, and you and your provider can collaborate to find solutions.

Utilizing technology in healthcare can significantly enhance communication. Digital health records and patient portals are valuable tools for sharing information with your healthcare team. These resources allow you to access your medical history, check test results, and reach out to providers between appointments. For example, if you have a question about a recent lab result, you can send a secure message through the portal and often receive a quicker response than waiting for your next visit. Many systems also offer online appointment scheduling, making it easier to coordinate your care.

Access to these technological resources streamlines communication and gives you greater control over your health. When you can review your own medical information, you're better equipped to make informed decisions and engage in more meaningful conversations with your healthcare providers. This approach is particularly beneficial for those managing chronic conditions, as it supports timely adjustments to treatment plans and quick responses to new issues.

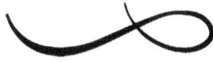

Chapter 27: Financial Tips for Managing Chronic Conditions

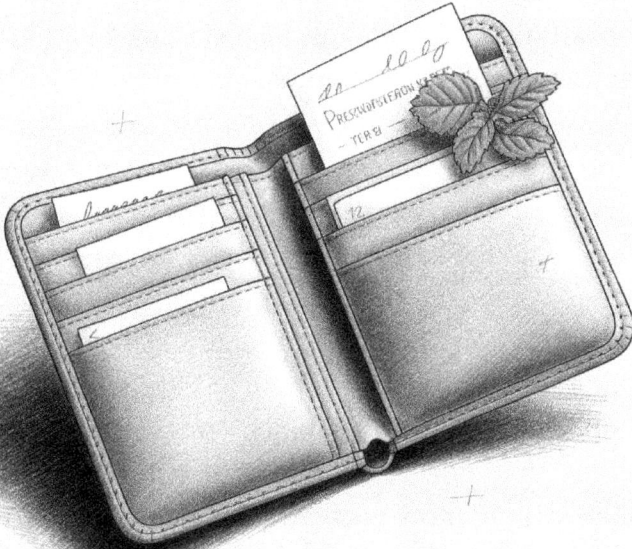

Managing the financial aspects of chronic conditions like **diabetes**, **hypertension**, and **musculoskeletal disorders** can often feel complex and overwhelming. However, with careful planning and decisions grounded in solid data, you can keep expenses in check while ensuring high-quality care. Begin by thoroughly reviewing your insurance options to grasp the details of each health plan. Compare them by examining:

- Monthly premiums
- Co-pays
- Deductibles
- The range of covered services

Prioritize plans that offer comprehensive coverage, including preventive care and necessary specialist visits, to help minimize out-of-pocket costs. This strategy not only secures access to essential healthcare services but also supports you in managing long-term financial responsibilities.

Prescription medications can quickly become a significant expense, but there are several strategies to help reduce these costs. Opting for *generic options*, which are just as effective as brand-name versions but much more affordable, is one possibility. Discuss with your healthcare provider the potential for switching to these budget-friendly alternatives. Additionally, explore pharmaceutical assistance programs from various organizations that offer substantial discounts on prescription drugs, making them more accessible for those managing chronic conditions.

Community resources and non-profit organizations provide valuable support in reducing healthcare expenses. Many local health departments and community clinics offer low-cost screenings, consultations, and educational workshops tailored for individuals with chronic conditions. These services deliver essential information and support, empowering you to manage your health more effectively while alleviating financial pressure.

Expenses related to dietary management can accumulate quickly, but smart planning can help you maintain a healthy diet without overspending. Consider the following strategies:

- Purchase seasonal produce
- Buy items in bulk
- Plan meals carefully to minimize food waste

Consulting with a registered dietitian can also be very beneficial. They can collaborate with you to create meal plans that align with your budget and dietary needs, ensuring you receive the necessary nutrients to manage your condition.

Technology and telehealth services have transformed how people access healthcare, providing a more affordable alternative to traditional in-person visits. Many providers now offer virtual consultations, which can lower travel costs and save time, making it easier to receive care from the comfort of your home.

Staying active is essential for managing chronic conditions, and it doesn't have to be expensive. Consider affordable options like walking, exercising at home, or joining community fitness classes. These activities often cost less than gym memberships but still support your health and help manage symptoms effectively.

Regularly checking your medical bills and insurance statements is crucial to catch errors and avoid unnecessary charges. Pay close attention to any mistakes or inconsistencies, and don't hesitate to contact billing departments if you need clarification. If paying bills becomes challenging, inquire about payment plans that can help you manage costs without compromising the quality of care.

Setting aside money for future healthcare expenses is another important aspect of managing costs. Think about contributing to **Health Savings Accounts (HSAs)** or **Flexible Spending Accounts (FSAs)**, which allow you to save pre-tax dollars for medical needs and provide a financial cushion for future healthcare spending.

Understanding your financial rights and protections under healthcare laws is vital. Stay informed about policy changes that could impact costs or access to services for chronic disease management. This knowledge empowers you to make informed decisions and advocate effectively for your healthcare needs.

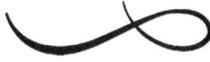

Chapter 28: Reliable Sources for Chronic Disease Management

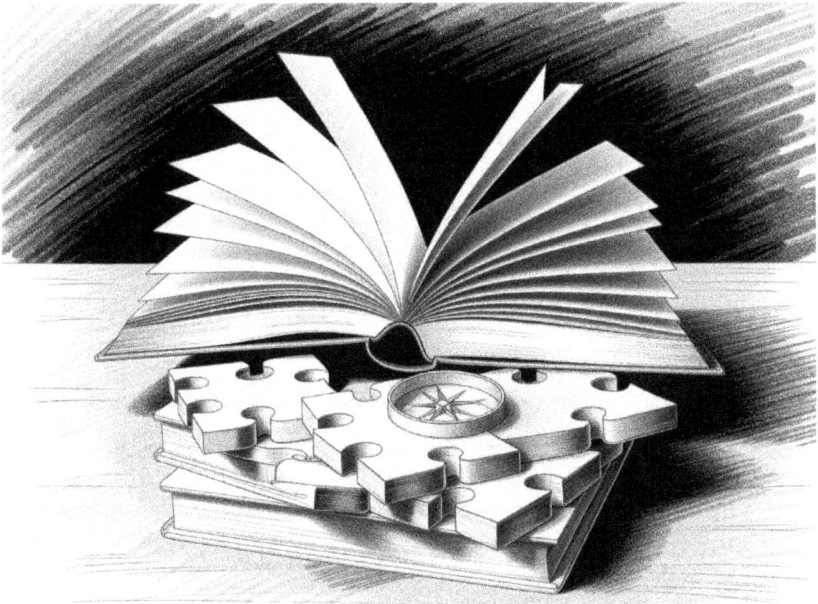

In today's digital age, effectively managing chronic diseases involves a solid understanding of your specific condition and access to trustworthy information sources. The internet is filled with resources, but it's crucial to evaluate which ones you can rely on. Government health websites, like the **Centers for Disease Control and Prevention (CDC)** and the **National Institutes of Health (NIH)**, are excellent starting points. These sites offer evidence-based guidelines and the latest updates on various health conditions, ensuring that the information you access is both accurate and up-to-date.

For instance, the CDC provides extensive resources on managing chronic diseases such as *diabetes* and *hypertension*. Their guidelines are crafted by experts in the field and are regularly updated to reflect the latest research findings. The NIH also offers a wealth of information on health topics, including in-depth analyses of musculoskeletal disorders, helping you find scientifically validated content that can guide your daily management strategies.

Reliable medical organizations provide specialized information tailored to specific conditions. Consider the following organizations:

- The**American Diabetes Association**offers resources that cover dietary guidelines, exercise recommendations, and the latest advancements in diabetes management. Their website features tools for tracking blood glucose levels and medication adherence, which are essential for individuals living with diabetes.
- The**American Heart Association**focuses on cardiovascular health and lifestyle changes for those managing hypertension.
- The**Arthritis Foundation**provides detailed guidance on pain management and strategies to improve mobility for individuals facing musculoskeletal challenges.

Health apps and digital platforms play a significant role in managing chronic conditions. Applications like **MyFitnessPal** and **Healthline** include features for tracking symptoms, medication schedules, and lifestyle changes. MyFitnessPal allows users to log daily food intake and exercise routines, offering insights into how these factors impact overall health. Healthline provides various tools, such as symptom checkers and medication reminders, which can help you stay on track with your health management plan.

Subscribing to newsletters from reputable health organizations is another effective way to stay informed. These newsletters often feature the latest research findings, practical tips for managing your condition, and updates on emerging treatments. Regular updates help ensure that your management strategies align with the most current medical guidelines.

Online forums and support groups can be incredibly beneficial, providing opportunities to share experiences and gather insights from others managing similar conditions. It's important to choose forums moderated by healthcare professionals to ensure the credibility of the information shared. Connecting with a community of individuals who understand your challenges can offer both emotional support and practical advice, enhancing your ability to manage your condition effectively.

When evaluating online resources, verify the credibility of the information by checking the qualifications of the authors and the sources cited in articles and publications. Reputable websites typically list the credentials of their contributors, allowing you to confirm their expertise. Look for articles that reference peer-reviewed studies or guidelines from recognized health organizations, as these are strong indicators of reliable information.

Workshops, webinars, and seminars are fantastic ways to stay informed about the latest research findings and management strategies for chronic diseases. Organized by hospitals, universities, and community health centers, these educational opportunities provide access to expert knowledge and the most current information in the field. By attending these events, you gain valuable insights into emerging treatment options, evidence-based lifestyle modifications, and technological innovations that can enhance the management of conditions like **diabetes, hypertension,** and **musculoskeletal disorders**. Many sessions include interactive components, allowing you to ask questions and engage directly with experts, which deepens your understanding and offers practical advice tailored to your health needs.

Health fairs and community events are excellent resources for individuals managing chronic conditions. These gatherings typically feature complimentary health screenings, educational materials, and expert presentations, making them both accessible and informative. Participating in these events allows you to gather important information about your health status through screenings and receive personalized advice from healthcare professionals. Additionally, these events help connect you with local resources and support networks, which are vital for ongoing health management.

Building a network with healthcare professionals is essential for receiving personalized advice and staying informed about new treatment options and lifestyle recommendations. Connect with:

- Pharmacists, who can clarify medication management, including potential interactions and side effects.
- Dietitians, who assist in developing nutrition plans that align with your health goals.
- Physical therapists, who create exercise regimens to enhance mobility and alleviate pain, particularly for those with musculoskeletal issues.

Maintaining these relationships fosters a support system that offers ongoing advice and necessary adjustments to your care plan.

Consider enrolling in chronic disease self-management programs, which offer structured guidance and peer support to empower individuals with tools and strategies for effective condition management. Participants learn about goal setting, problem-solving, and decision-making skills that are crucial for daily management. The peer support aspect connects you with others facing similar challenges, creating a sense of community and shared learning. This environment encourages motivation and helps you stay committed to your health goals.

A personal health journal is a practical tool for documenting new information, tracking health metrics, and evaluating the effectiveness of management strategies. Recording details such as *blood sugar levels*, *blood pressure readings*, and *physical activity* helps identify patterns and make informed decisions about your care. This journal becomes a valuable resource during medical appointments, allowing you to share accurate and comprehensive information with your healthcare providers. Reviewing entries helps determine which strategies are effective and where adjustments may be needed, supporting continuous improvement in health management.

Regular discussions with healthcare providers about recent advancements are crucial for keeping your care plan up to date. Engage with your doctors to discuss new research findings, treatment options, and lifestyle recommendations that could enhance your condition management. Staying informed and open to new ideas ensures your management plan remains current and effective. These conversations also demonstrate your commitment to health and help build a collaborative relationship with your healthcare team.

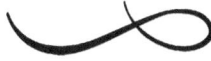

Chapter 29: Creating Your Personalized Daily Management Plan

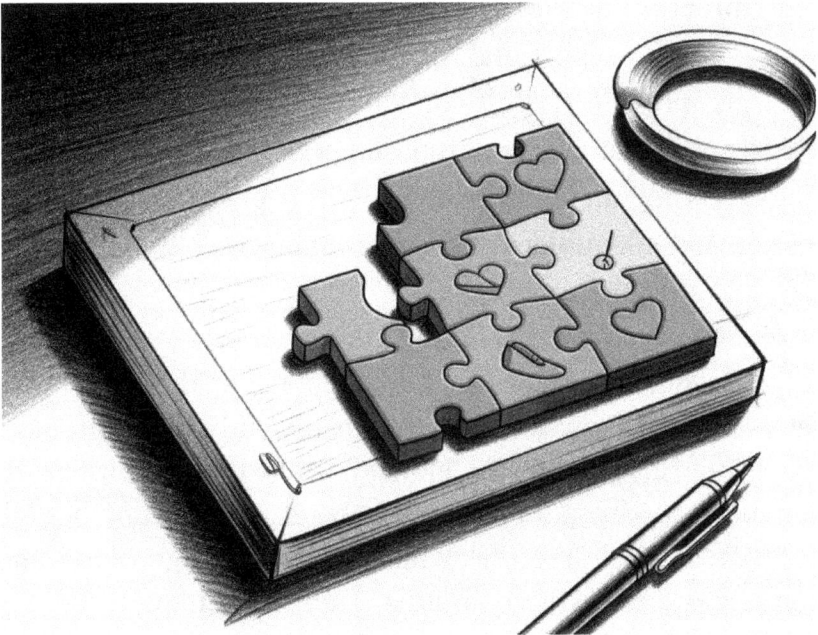

Tip

Start your health journal today by recording your daily symptoms, medication, meals, and activity. Even brief notes can reveal important patterns over time, helping you

*and your healthcare team make better decisions. Use a
notebook or a health app—whichever fits your lifestyle best.
Consistency is more important than perfection, so don't
worry if you miss a day. Your journal is a powerful tool for
tracking progress and staying motivated on your journey.*

Managing a chronic condition begins with a comprehensive assessment of your health status. This process includes gathering and analyzing recent medical reports, personal observations, and insights from healthcare providers. By taking these steps, you can identify specific areas that require attention, such as monitoring blood sugar levels for diabetes, tracking blood pressure readings for hypertension, or implementing pain management strategies for musculoskeletal issues.

Start with your most recent medical reports, as these documents offer a detailed overview of your health and essential data on various metrics crucial for managing chronic conditions. For instance, individuals living with diabetes may find *hemoglobin A1c* levels in their reports, which reflect average blood sugar over the past two to three months. Those with hypertension will typically see detailed blood pressure readings over time, including systolic and diastolic values. People dealing with musculoskeletal issues might discover information on joint health, inflammation markers, or imaging results. Reviewing these reports with your healthcare provider can clarify your current health status and highlight areas that may need improvement.

Personal observations are also vital in assessing health. Pay attention to your daily well-being and note any symptoms or changes in your condition. For example, someone with diabetes might notice fluctuations in energy levels, episodes of hypoglycemia, or changes in vision. Individuals with hypertension may experience headaches, dizziness, or fatigue, while those with musculoskeletal issues could report varying levels of pain, stiffness, or mobility challenges. Keeping a daily log of these observations can help you understand how your condition impacts daily life and assist in identifying patterns or triggers.

Input from healthcare providers is another essential component of the assessment. Regular check-ups with your primary care physician, endocrinologist, cardiologist, or other specialists provide expert guidance on managing your condition. These professionals help interpret medical reports, offer personalized advice on lifestyle changes, and recommend specific treatments or interventions. Maintaining open communication with your healthcare team gives you a well-rounded understanding of your health and the steps needed to enhance it.

Once you have a clear picture of your health status, set realistic and achievable goals that align with your needs, lifestyle, and personal priorities. Establish both short-term and long-term objectives that are measurable and time-bound. For example, if managing hypertension, a short-term goal could be lowering blood pressure by a specific number of points within three months. A long-term goal might involve consistently maintaining a healthy blood pressure level over the next year.

Utilize the **SMART** criteria when setting goals:

- Specific: Clearly define what you want to accomplish, such as reducing daily sugar intake to a certain number of grams.
- Measurable: Allow you to track progress, like aiming to walk 10,000 steps a day or complete a set number of strength training sessions each week.
- Achievable: Ensure goals are realistic and attainable, considering your current health status and available resources.
- Relevant: Support your overall health objectives, such as improving cardiovascular health or managing weight.
- Time-bound: Have a clear deadline, which helps keep you motivated.

Document your goals in a personal health journal to track progress and make adjustments as needed. This journal captures your efforts, achievements, and challenges. Regularly reviewing your goals and reflecting on your progress helps maintain motivation and focus on your health objectives. It also serves as a valuable resource for discussions with healthcare providers, enabling them to offer tailored advice and support.

A structured daily routine is essential for effectively managing chronic conditions like **diabetes**, **hypertension**, and **musculoskeletal disorders**. This plan should be customized to fit your unique health needs and lifestyle, ensuring it remains both practical and sustainable. Begin by identifying the most important management strategies for your condition and gradually weave them into your daily schedule.

For those managing diabetes, establishing a consistent schedule for checking blood glucose is crucial. Aim to monitor your blood sugar at specific times each day, such as before meals and at bedtime. Utilize a calibrated glucose meter and keep a detailed log of your readings to spot trends and make informed decisions about your food and medication. Focus on planning balanced meals with controlled carbohydrates, emphasizing:

- whole grains
- lean proteins
- a variety of vegetables

Preparing meals in advance can help you stick to healthier choices and steer clear of less nutritious options.

Incorporating physical activity is another vital component of diabetes management. Strive for at least 150 minutes of moderate-intensity aerobic exercise each week, which can be broken down into 30-minute sessions on most days. Activities like brisk walking, cycling, and swimming are all effective, as regular exercise enhances insulin sensitivity and supports weight management. Choose workout times that suit your energy levels and daily commitments, whether that's a morning jog or an evening yoga class.

Managing hypertension also involves effective stress control, so consider including activities like yoga, meditation, or deep-breathing exercises in your daily routine. These practices can help lower blood pressure and improve overall well-being. Focus on a low-sodium diet to support heart health by planning meals around fresh, unprocessed foods and using herbs and spices for flavor instead of salt. Keep an eye on your sodium intake and aim to stay within the recommended limit of **2,300 mg** per day or less, as advised by your healthcare provider.

Regular exercise is beneficial for those with high blood pressure as well. Aerobic activities such as walking, jogging, or cycling can help lower blood pressure and enhance cardiovascular health. Incorporate strength training two to three times a week to further boost your fitness. Consistency is key, so choose activities you enjoy and can sustain over time.

For individuals with musculoskeletal disorders, daily exercises that promote flexibility and strength are essential. Tailor your routine to match your physical abilities and pain levels, focusing on low-impact activities that protect your joints. Stretching helps maintain flexibility, while strength training supports muscle health and joint stability. Collaborating with a physical therapist can help you develop a personalized exercise plan that aligns with your needs and limitations.

A flexible daily routine allows you to navigate unexpected changes or challenges. Life doesn't always go as planned, so being adaptable is important for maintaining healthy habits without feeling overwhelmed. If a meeting runs late and delays your meal, keep healthy snacks on hand to help stabilize your blood sugar. If you miss your usual workout, consider a shorter session or opt for another activity that fits your schedule.

Incorporating technology into your daily management plan can significantly improve your ability to monitor and manage chronic conditions. Health apps offer practical tools for tracking specific metrics, setting medication reminders, and monitoring symptoms in real time. These applications can be tailored to meet your individual needs, allowing you to log essential data such as:

- **blood glucose levels**
- **blood pressure readings**
- **pain intensity**

Maintaining a consistent record of this information helps you identify trends over time, guiding your healthcare decisions and any necessary adjustments to your management strategy. Many apps also include goal-setting and progress-tracking features, which can help you stay motivated and focused on your health objectives.

Local community resources are invaluable for providing support and encouragement. Many areas have structured support groups specifically designed for individuals managing chronic conditions. These groups create a welcoming space to share personal experiences, exchange practical advice, and receive emotional support from others who truly understand your situation. Engaging in these groups can foster a sense of connection and accountability, reinforcing your commitment to your management plan.

Exercise classes tailored for those with chronic conditions are another excellent resource. Led by trained professionals who understand the unique needs and limitations associated with chronic diseases, these classes guide you through safe and effective exercises. Regular participation can enhance your fitness, alleviate symptoms, and improve your overall well-being.

A strong support network is crucial for effectively managing chronic disease. Family, friends, and healthcare providers can offer encouragement, share their experiences, and provide assistance when needed. Keeping communication open with your support system ensures they understand your health goals and can help you stay on track. Share your management plan, discuss your progress, and invite their input and advice. Collaborating in this way strengthens your resolve and provides the emotional and practical support necessary to navigate the challenges of managing a chronic condition.

Open communication within your support network involves being honest about your needs and challenges. Regularly updating family and friends on your progress and any difficulties you encounter allows them to offer targeted support and helps prevent misunderstandings. Stay connected with healthcare providers by sharing your health data, discussing any changes in your condition, and seeking their advice on adjustments to your management plan. Being proactive in this manner keeps your care aligned with your health goals and ensures it adapts to any changes in your condition.

Online communities and forums dedicated to chronic disease management can also provide valuable connections. These platforms connect you with individuals from diverse backgrounds who face similar challenges. Engaging in these communities can offer new perspectives, practical tips, and a sense of camaraderie. Always verify the credibility of information shared in these forums and consult healthcare professionals before making significant changes to your management plan.

To manage chronic conditions effectively, it's essential to prioritize regular reviews and evaluations of your daily management plan. Consider using a health journal to systematically record daily metrics such as specific blood sugar readings (for example, *fasting* and *postprandial* levels), blood pressure measurements (like morning and evening readings), or pain scores on a scale of 1 to 10. In addition to these quantitative measures, include detailed notes about your physical symptoms and emotional state to create a comprehensive picture of your health. This thorough documentation helps you spot trends and patterns over time, making it easier to identify areas that might need adjustments or improvements.

Careful review of health data plays a key role in determining how well the management plan is working. Look for specific patterns in your metrics that could signal a need for change. For instance, if you notice consistently high blood sugar levels at certain times, it may be time to reconsider your meal schedule or medication dosages. If blood pressure tends to rise during stressful periods, try incorporating stress-reduction techniques such as mindfulness exercises or breathing practices into your daily routine. Recognizing these trends empowers you to make informed decisions about possible changes to your management plan.

Regular appointments with healthcare professionals are vital for keeping the plan effective and aligned with your health goals.

Schedule consistent check-ins with your primary care physician or relevant specialists to discuss your progress. Bring your health journal to these meetings so your healthcare team can gain a full understanding of your condition and offer tailored advice and recommendations. They can help interpret your data, suggest changes to your treatment plan, and share new strategies to enhance your quality of life.

Staying updated with new research or treatment options is also important for managing chronic conditions. The medical field is always evolving, with new studies and innovations emerging frequently. Stay informed by subscribing to newsletters from trusted health organizations, attending workshops, or joining webinars. Keeping current with the latest developments helps you learn about new treatments or management strategies that could benefit your condition. Being open to trying new approaches or updating your current plan can make a significant difference in managing symptoms and improving overall well-being.

Flexibility and adaptability are crucial when dealing with chronic conditions. As you gather more data and insights, be prepared to adjust your management plan as needed. This could mean changing your diet, updating your exercise routine, or considering new medication options. Approach these changes with an open mind and a willingness to explore different solutions. What works for one person may not work for another, so it's important to find the strategies that best fit your individual needs and lifestyle.

Feedback from your support network can provide valuable perspectives. Family members, friends, and healthcare providers may offer insights you haven't considered. Engage in conversations about your management plan and remain open to their suggestions. Their support and encouragement can help you stay motivated and committed to your health goals.

Daily Self-Care Routines for Disease Management

A structured morning routine is essential for effectively managing chronic conditions like **diabetes**, **hypertension**, and **musculoskeletal disorders**. This approach not only sets a positive tone for the day but also helps you address your specific health needs right from the start.

Begin each morning with a self-assessment to gauge your physical and emotional state. Take a few moments to reflect on how you feel and whether any new symptoms have emerged, such as increased pain or changes in energy levels. Jot down these details in your health journal, noting specifics like intensity and duration. Tracking this information can help you identify patterns over time, provide valuable insights to your healthcare provider, and enable you to adjust your daily goals and tasks to align with your current condition. For instance, if you notice you're feeling more fatigued than usual, you might choose to reduce your exercise or allow yourself extra time to rest.

Review your daily goals and tasks to maintain a sense of control and purpose. Clearly outline what you want to achieve, whether it's related to work, personal projects, or health management. Be open to adjusting these objectives as needed to accommodate any changes in your condition or schedule. Staying flexible empowers you to respond to your body's needs without feeling overwhelmed.

Prepare all necessary medications, devices, and supplies before starting your day. Ensure that your **glucometer** or **blood pressure monitor** is functioning properly and that you have enough test strips or medication for the day ahead. Keeping these items organized in a designated spot can streamline your morning routine and reduce stress, as having everything ready minimizes the risk of overlooking important self-care steps.

Nutrition and hydration are vital for managing chronic conditions. Kick off your day with a balanced breakfast that aligns with your health requirements. For diabetes, this might involve selecting complex carbohydrates, proteins, and healthy fats to help stabilize blood sugar levels. If you're managing hypertension, focus on low-sodium options to support heart health. Planning and preparing meals in advance can help you adhere to dietary recommendations. Strategies like batch cooking or pre-portioning ingredients can save time and simplify following your meal plan.

Staying hydrated is equally important. Aim for at least eight 8-ounce glasses of water each day, adjusting this amount based on your health needs and your provider's advice. Proper hydration supports overall health and can help alleviate symptoms related to chronic conditions.

Incorporating physical activity into your morning routine is crucial for effective disease management. Choose exercises that align with your health goals and physical abilities. Consider the following options:

- A 30-minute walk
- Yoga
- Light strength training

These activities can provide significant benefits, enhancing both physical health and mental clarity while reducing stress. If you have musculoskeletal limitations, feel free to adapt your exercises—using resistance bands instead of weights or focusing on low-impact activities like swimming or cycling can be beneficial.

Mindfulness or meditation practices can further enhance your health management efforts. These techniques help reduce stress and improve mental clarity, which is especially important for conditions like hypertension or musculoskeletal discomfort. Spend a few minutes concentrating on your breath or following a guided meditation to set a positive tone for the day and build resilience for any challenges that may come your way.

Midday monitoring is essential for effectively managing chronic conditions. Around lunchtime, take a moment to measure key health indicators like **blood glucose levels** or **systolic and diastolic blood pressure**. This practice gives you a clear snapshot of your current health status and empowers you to make informed decisions about any necessary adjustments. For example, if your blood glucose level is above the target range, consider modifying your meal plan by incorporating more *fiber-rich foods* such as whole grains and vegetables, or adjusting your medication dosage as advised by your healthcare provider. If your blood pressure readings exceed the recommended levels, try a brief relaxation exercise like deep breathing or meditation, or reduce your sodium intake for the rest of the day. Be sure to record these readings in your health journal to track patterns over time and facilitate discussions with your healthcare team.

A short rest period in the afternoon can be particularly beneficial for those experiencing musculoskeletal discomfort. A quick nap or some relaxation can help restore energy and alleviate fatigue, which often intensifies with chronic pain. Even just 15 to 20 minutes of rest can significantly improve how you feel for the rest of the day. Use this time to practice *mindfulness techniques* or simply close your eyes and unwind, allowing your body a chance to recover.

Social and emotional well-being are vital components in managing chronic diseases. Engaging in social activities or connecting with others provides valuable emotional support and helps diminish feelings of isolation. You might consider:

- Scheduling a phone call with a friend
- Joining an online support group to share experiences
- Spending time with family for comfort and motivation

These interactions not only lift your mood but also foster a sense of community and belonging, both of which are crucial for mental health.

Incorporating stress-reducing techniques into your afternoon routine can enhance your emotional well-being. **Deep breathing exercises**, **progressive muscle relaxation**, or **guided imagery** can help lower stress levels and improve mental clarity. These straightforward practices assist in managing stress, benefiting your overall health and supporting chronic condition management. Dedicate a few minutes each day to these exercises to help yourself unwind and regain focus.

As the day winds down, take some time for evening reflection and planning. Review your health journal entries to assess how effective your daily routine has been. Identify what worked well and where you might need to make adjustments. This reflection helps refine your management plan and fosters a sense of accomplishment and progress. Celebrate your successes, no matter how small, and let them inspire you to keep moving forward.

Preparing for the next day is a key part of your evening routine. Organize your medication doses so they are ready and easy to access. Plan your meals and activities, making any necessary adjustments based on your health metrics. Creating a restful sleep environment is crucial for overall health and symptom management. Establish a consistent bedtime routine that promotes relaxation, such as reading a book or listening to calming music. Ensure your sleep space is comfortable and free from distractions, as quality sleep is essential for both physical and mental recovery.

Sample Action Plan Templates for Daily Self-Management

A personalized action plan template is essential for effectively managing chronic conditions. This framework helps you organize daily activities, monitor specific health metrics, and track your progress over time. The goal is to create a plan that is both adaptable and comprehensive, allowing for adjustments to address various chronic issues such as **diabetes**, **hypertension**, and **musculoskeletal disorders**.

Start with a section for daily goals that are specific, measurable, and directly linked to your overall health objectives. For example, someone managing diabetes might aim to keep blood glucose levels between 70 and 130 mg/dL before meals. For hypertension, a goal could be to engage in 30 minutes of moderate-intensity aerobic exercise, like brisk walking or cycling, at least five days a week. Clearly defining these objectives sharpens your focus and enhances motivation.

Include a section for self-care tasks that outlines daily activities essential for managing your condition. For diabetes, this could involve following meal planning strategies such as counting carbohydrates and timing insulin doses. For musculoskeletal disorders, this section might detail targeted exercises to improve joint flexibility and strength. Providing detailed prompts and examples in this part of the template can help you identify the most relevant tasks for your situation.

The template should also feature a section for monitoring activities, specifying which health metrics to track each day. Individuals with hypertension, for instance, should measure blood pressure at least twice daily. Those with diabetes need to check blood glucose levels several times a day, especially before and after meals. Keeping consistent records of these metrics makes it easier to identify trends and make informed decisions about your health management.

A space for reflection notes adds value to the template. Here, you can jot down thoughts and observations about your health management, analyze which strategies were effective, note any obstacles, and record how you felt physically and emotionally throughout the day. These reflections can provide insights into your progress and help you adjust your plan as needed.

To make the action plan effective, tailor it to your needs by first identifying specific health goals. These might include lowering systolic blood pressure to below 130 mmHg or increasing weekly physical activity to at least 150 minutes. Listing unique health challenges, such as medication side effects or dietary restrictions, along with your motivations, helps you stay focused on what matters most.

A self-management routine should be flexible, as health status and lifestyle can change. Your action plan should adapt to these shifts. For example, if musculoskeletal pain flares up, you might switch to low-impact activities like swimming or yoga. If your healthcare provider prescribes a new medication or treatment, be sure to update your plan to reflect these changes.

Visual aids such as color-coding or symbols can make your template easier to navigate. You might assign colors to indicate priority tasks or highlight areas that need immediate attention. A red symbol could mark urgent tasks, while a green one might indicate completed activities. These visual cues help you stay focused on the most important aspects of your health management.

To effectively integrate your action plan into daily life, begin by breaking down each task into clear, manageable steps. Establish a morning routine that directly supports your health goals, such as checking **blood glucose** or taking prescribed medications at set times. Consider using digital tools like smartphone apps to set reminders for these tasks, making them a regular part of your schedule. These applications can also help you track progress with visual feedback and notifications that reinforce your routine. If you prefer not to use digital tools, a physical planner or calendar can effectively organize daily tasks and allow you to mark them off as you complete them.

Reach out to family or friends for support by sharing your health goals and asking for their encouragement or assistance. For example, a family member might join you for a daily walk, or a friend could remind you to take your medication on time. This support system not only strengthens your commitment but also provides emotional backing, helping to ease feelings of isolation.

Regularly review your action plan to monitor progress and make any necessary adjustments. Set aside time each week to look over health metrics, such as **blood pressure** or pain levels, and compare them to your goals. Record any changes or patterns you notice, and use this information to refine your strategies. If a particular approach isn't working, feel free to change it as needed. This ongoing process helps build positive habits and address setbacks, ensuring your plan remains effective and relevant to your needs.

To assess how well your plan is working, focus on measurable results. Ask yourself questions like:

- Are my symptoms improving?
- Is my quality of life better?
- Am I meeting my health goals?

Use specific criteria, such as lower blood pressure or improved mobility, to gauge progress. If you identify areas that need improvement, pinpoint possible obstacles and brainstorm practical solutions. This might involve adjusting your exercise routine, exploring different dietary options, or consulting your doctor for additional advice.

Healthcare providers play a crucial role in refining your plan. Bring your progress notes to medical appointments and discuss your findings with your provider. Collaborating ensures your approach aligns with medical recommendations and allows for adjustments based on professional advice. Healthcare professionals can suggest new treatments or strategies to enhance management, and their expertise, combined with your observations, creates a solid foundation for handling chronic disease.

Regular self-reflection is key to staying motivated and committed. Check in with yourself about your emotional and mental well-being, as these factors significantly impact your ability to manage a chronic condition. Ask yourself questions like:

- How do I feel about my progress?

- What emotional challenges am I facing?
- Am I experiencing stress or anxiety related to my condition?

Reflecting on these questions helps you understand the psychological aspects of disease management and supports a more holistic approach.

Incorporate stress-relief activities into your routine, such as *meditation* or *journaling*, to bolster your mental health. These practices can help reduce stress, bring clarity, and improve focus, making it easier to adhere to your action plan. Managing a chronic condition requires ongoing effort, so be sure to treat yourself with compassion. Celebrate small successes and acknowledge the daily work you put into your health.

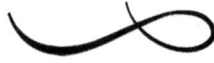

Chapter 30: Sustaining Health and Quality of Life Long-Term

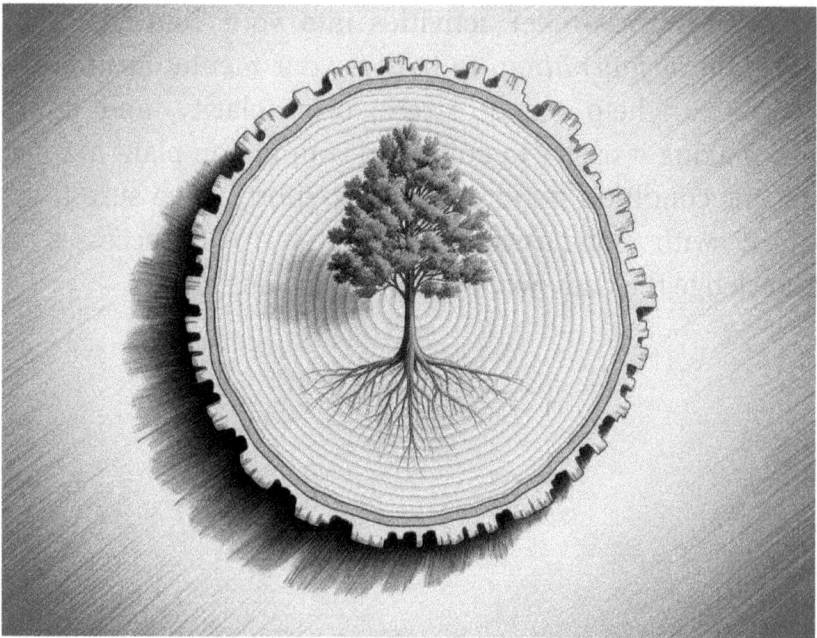

Tip

Start small and build gradually—this is the secret to making healthy habits stick. Instead of overhauling your entire routine, choose one manageable change, like adding a daily walk or prepping meals in advance. As these actions become second nature, you'll find it easier to add more. This approach prevents burnout and fits better into a busy lifestyle, making long-term health management more achievable and less overwhelming.

S ustainable habits are essential for effectively managing chronic diseases over the long haul. Achieving success hinges on selecting practices that are both enjoyable and manageable, allowing them to seamlessly blend into your daily life rather than feeling like burdens. This strategy helps prevent burnout, which often arises when people try to implement drastic changes too quickly. By making gradual adjustments that resonate with personal preferences and current lifestyles, you significantly boost your chances of sticking with these habits.

A practical way to cultivate lasting habits is to concentrate on small, consistent actions that fit into your existing routine. This approach makes it easier to adopt and maintain new behaviors. For example, if you're looking to enhance your diet, consider adding an extra serving of *vegetables* to your meals each day. This straightforward step can gradually lead to a more balanced diet without becoming overwhelming. If your goal is to increase physical activity, start with a brief daily walk around your neighborhood. Once this becomes a regular part of your day, you can gradually extend the duration or intensity of your exercise.

A balanced diet is a cornerstone of sustainable health practices. Consuming a variety of foods that provide essential nutrients— like fruits, vegetables, whole grains, lean proteins, and healthy fats—supports overall well-being. Preparing meals in advance ensures you have nutritious options available throughout the week, reducing the temptation to opt for less healthy choices. Dedicating a few hours each week to meal prep can save time and make it easier to stick to healthy selections.

Regular physical activity is vital for long-term health management. Establishing a consistent exercise routine can significantly enhance well-being and help manage chronic conditions. Choose activities you enjoy that fit your schedule, whether it's morning yoga, an evening jog, or a weekend hike. The key is to find something you look forward to and can easily incorporate into your daily life. Committing to a regular exercise schedule, such as:

- A 30-minute workout three times a week
- Morning yoga sessions
- Evening jogs or weekend hikes

helps you stay accountable and makes physical activity a natural part of your routine.

Managing stress is equally important for maintaining sustainable health habits. Chronic stress can exacerbate symptoms of many conditions, so discovering effective coping strategies is crucial. Mindfulness practices like meditation or deep breathing exercises can be integrated into your daily routine to help alleviate stress and enhance mental clarity. Even dedicating just a few minutes each day to mindfulness can lead to noticeable improvements in overall well-being.

Community and support systems are vital for sustaining healthy habits. Engaging with local groups, online communities, or wellness programs can provide the motivation and accountability needed to stay focused on your health goals. These support networks foster a sense of belonging and encouragement, making it easier to maintain your habits. Consider joining a local exercise class, participating in an online forum with others who share your health objectives, or attending wellness workshops in your area. These interactions offer valuable insights, shared experiences, and support, all of which contribute to maintaining health improvements over time.

Adaptability is a key element of effective health management, particularly when navigating chronic conditions. Life can throw unexpected challenges our way, so it's essential to adjust health strategies to meet new circumstances. For example, if longer work hours disrupt your usual exercise routine, consider switching to shorter, high-intensity workouts that can fit into a 20-30 minute window. When family responsibilities take up more of your time, choose meals that can be prepared in under 30 minutes, utilizing pre-chopped vegetables or meal-prepping on less busy days to help you stay on track with your dietary needs. This flexible approach ensures that health management remains a priority, even when life gets hectic.

Resilience is crucial in managing chronic diseases, as it involves developing coping skills to handle setbacks and maintain a positive outlook during challenging times. Breaking down larger health goals into smaller, manageable tasks makes them feel more achievable and provides frequent opportunities to recognize and celebrate your progress, which can enhance motivation and morale. For instance, if your goal is to lower blood pressure, start by focusing on reducing sodium intake by 1,000 mg per day and take a moment to acknowledge your success when you reach that milestone. Viewing challenges as opportunities for growth can transform setbacks into valuable lessons, and each obstacle you overcome showcases your strength and adaptability, reinforcing your ability to manage your condition effectively.

Clear communication with healthcare providers is essential for keeping health management strategies effective and current. Regular check-ins with your healthcare team allow you to discuss any changes in your condition, review your current plan, and make necessary adjustments. Taking the initiative to seek advice can help prevent minor health issues from escalating into major problems. For example, if you notice changes in symptoms or a new treatment isn't working as expected, don't hesitate to reach out to your provider right away. They can suggest adjustments or offer insights you might not have considered.

Keeping a detailed record of health metrics and experiences can make conversations with your healthcare team more productive. Bring your health journal to appointments to provide a clear picture of your progress, including specific data like blood pressure readings, weight changes, or adherence to your diet. This practice helps your provider understand your situation better and empowers you to take a more active role in managing your health.

When your healthcare provider offers feedback, incorporate those suggestions into your daily routine to maintain effective management strategies. If you receive a new exercise plan or dietary advice, introduce these changes gradually and monitor how they impact your health metrics. Adjusting your plan in this way helps ensure it aligns with your health goals and fits seamlessly into your lifestyle.

A comprehensive lifestyle approach is essential for managing chronic diseases, as it addresses the physical, mental, and emotional aspects of health. When you make improvements in one area, it often leads to positive changes in others, creating a ripple effect that enhances your overall well-being. For example, regular physical activity not only boosts **muscle strength** and supports **cardiovascular health** but also sharpens **cognitive abilities** and promotes **emotional stability**. Achieving emotional balance can help reduce stress, which may lower blood pressure and support better glycemic control.

To nurture your mental and emotional health, engage in activities that bring you joy and relaxation. Hobbies like painting, gardening, or playing a musical instrument provide creative outlets and foster a sense of accomplishment. These activities can help distract you from daily stressors while stimulating cognitive functions, benefiting your brain health. Building and maintaining social connections is also vital. Regular interactions with friends, family, or community groups offer emotional support and help alleviate feelings of loneliness. Consider the following options to enhance your sense of belonging and community:

- Scheduling a weekly coffee with a friend
- Joining a local club
- Participating in community events

If stress or emotional challenges feel overwhelming, reaching out to a professional is a smart choice. Licensed therapists or counselors can provide personalized strategies to manage stress, anxiety, or depression, which are common among those dealing with chronic conditions. Professional guidance introduces new coping methods and perspectives, supporting your emotional stability.

Staying balanced and prioritizing self-care are crucial for preventing burnout and supporting long-term well-being. Be aware of signs of burnout, such as ongoing fatigue, irritability, or lack of motivation, and take proactive steps to address them. Setting aside time each day for relaxation—whether it's reading, taking a bath, or enjoying quiet moments—helps maintain your energy and resilience for effective health management.

Complementary therapies can enhance conventional treatments and provide additional support for managing chronic diseases. **Yoga** and **meditation**, for instance, promote relaxation, increase flexibility, and sharpen mental focus. Yoga combines physical postures with breath control to reduce stress and build strength, while meditation encourages mindfulness and can be practiced almost anywhere, making it a practical tool for stress relief.

Acupuncture is another option for complementing standard treatments. This traditional practice uses fine needles placed at specific points on the body to stimulate healing and relieve pain. Research suggests it can help manage symptoms like pain or fatigue by activating the body's natural healing processes.

You can easily incorporate these complementary therapies into your routine without a significant time commitment. Even a few minutes of meditation each day or practicing yoga a couple of times a week can lead to noticeable improvements. The key is to find practices that resonate with you and integrate them into your daily life, allowing them to become lasting habits.

Setting long-term health and lifestyle goals is essential for effectively managing chronic conditions. These objectives should be both realistic and inspiring, providing a solid framework for ongoing health improvements. Start by clearly defining your aims, such as:

- Maintaining a target weight of 150 pounds
- Achieving a fitness level that allows you to run a 5K in under 30 minutes
- Adopting stress management techniques to reduce anxiety levels by half

Tools like vision boards or journals can help you visualize and articulate these aspirations. A vision board acts as a tangible reminder of your ambitions, filled with images and phrases that resonate with your health targets. Journals offer a structured way to document progress, track measurable results, and reflect on your experiences in detail.

Connecting your personal values to your health objectives is crucial for cultivating a strong sense of purpose and motivation.

When your goals align with what truly matters to you, they become more meaningful and easier to pursue. For example, if family is central to your life, you might aim to improve your cardiovascular fitness so you can join your children on weekend hikes. If creativity is important, maintaining your health could help sustain the energy needed for *painting* classes. Linking your aims to your values provides a compelling reason to stay committed, even when challenges arise.

Value-driven objectives enhance motivation and help you stick with your plans over time. For instance, committing to a weekly exercise routine allows you to enjoy hiking with your children, while following a meal plan can support your energy for creative pursuits like *painting*. These targets focus on improving your quality of life in personally meaningful ways, leading to a deeper sense of fulfillment and making the journey toward achieving them more rewarding.

Regularly reviewing your goals and making adjustments is important to keep them relevant and achievable. Life circumstances and priorities can shift, so your objectives should adapt accordingly. Set aside time every few months to assess whether your goals still align with your current situation and values. If they don't, take the initiative to update them. This flexibility allows you to remain open to new opportunities or challenges that may arise.

A new job that demands more of your time might require you to adjust your exercise schedule to fit a busier routine. On the other hand, discovering a newfound interest in cycling could inspire you to set a goal to train for a local cycling event. Staying flexible with your aims ensures that your health management strategies continue to support your well-being, even as life evolves.

To effectively track progress and make necessary adjustments, break each long-term goal into smaller, manageable steps. This approach makes larger objectives feel less daunting and provides regular milestones to celebrate. For example, if you want to lower your blood pressure, start by:

- Reducing your daily sodium intake by 1,500 mg
- Increasing your weekly physical activity to 150 minutes

Each small achievement reinforces your commitment and builds momentum toward your main goal.

Feedback from your support network can significantly enhance your journey. Share your objectives with family, friends, or healthcare professionals and invite their input. They can offer encouragement, help keep you accountable, and provide new perspectives you might not have considered. Collaborating in this way enriches your goal-setting process and strengthens your resolve to succeed.